Chakra Reading

&

Color Healing

Von Braschler

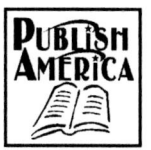

PublishAmerica
Baltimore

© 2005 by Von Braschler.
All rights reserved. No part of this book may be reproduced, stored in a retrieval system or transmitted in any form or by any means without the prior written permission of the publishers, except by a reviewer who may quote brief passages in a review to be printed in a newspaper, magazine or journal.

First printing

At the specific preference of the author, PublishAmerica allowed this work to remain exactly as the author intended, verbatim, without editorial input.

ISBN: 1-4137-7980-8
PUBLISHED BY PUBLISHAMERICA, LLLP
www.publishamerica.com
Baltimore

Printed in the United States of America

Dedicated to the
Theosophical Society

Table of Contents

Introduction 9

Chapter 1
Many Applications 14

Chapter 2
Basic Aura Reading and Energy Scanning 26

Chapter 3
Our Subtle Bodies 38

Chapter 4
Spotting Illness in Our Aura Energy Field 49

Chapter 5
Preparing for Energy Healing 65

Chapter 6
Healing Energy 76

Chapter 7
Various Modes and Techniques of Energy Healing 89

Chapter 8
The Magic Behind Energy Healing 107

Chapter 9
Stimulating Self-rejuvenation 117

Chapter 10
Treating the Subtle Illness, Based on Aura Reading 128

Chapter 11
Charting Progress with Follow-up Aura Reading 140

Chapter 12
The Role of the Wounded Healer 153

Chapter 13
Pets and Plants 165

Chapter 14
Practical Considerations for Energy Healers 176

Chapter 15
The Possible and the Impossible 182

Chapter 16
Reading Energy Levels All Around Us 192

Chapter 17
Exercises 199

Bibliography 218

Index 223

Thank you!

All personal after-tax profit from sale of this book will be donated by the author to animal charities for shelter, habitat, and protection. Thank you, readers, for helping to make this possible!

—Von Braschler

Introduction

Chakra reading combined with energy healing might sound incredibly difficult and magical to beginners, but that's only half true. The full truth is that energy healing that includes examination and changes to the chakras should not be difficult at all with proper orientation and practice. Anybody could do it. On the other hand, this holistic healing technique, while totally natural, is magical by definition. You see, energy healing that alters the chakras and aura involves transformation with the movement of energy at will. That's magic. We do this sort of natural magic all of the time without thinking much about it. Our thoughts, as energy waves, take shape and change the shapes of things when we send them. Our will exerts a mighty amount of personal energy that can be directed at something, when we know how to focus it and exercise it properly to bring about change. Furthermore, we can direct change with the energy that leaves our body, if we are able to focus it to bring about change. Energy in many forms is everywhere around us in nature and inside ourselves. The focused exercise of energy to transform, as with holistic healing, is natural magic. It is magic whereby we can access the mighty powers of nature all around us and work harmoniously with the divine within nature to bring about changes in our world. We can reshape our reality. We can work in harmony with the forces of nature to bring about health and needed change. This is natural magic that everyone can perform with the right orientation, focus, intent, and will. Everyone can learn to heal by learning to read the energy fields all around us—including the aura that radiates from the body. Once you learn to read the aura and interpret it with regard to health, you can transform the aura energetically by healing the illness that its colors and patterns indicate. The aura changes rapidly, providing almost instantaneous biofeedback of the energy healing that has occurred to the chakras as human energy centers.

Chakra healing, however, involves many levels of illness that can inflict and cripple any person, animal, or plant. This is because all life forms possess chakras as energy fields that reflect the many levels of their being. In this sense, we bear a striking resemblance to onions with their many layers of outer wrapping that collectively comprise the onion's total being. All living beings, including people, possess just as many layers of identity that comprise our total being. Most of these levels of our being, however, are so-called subtle bodies that exist outside of the physical body and, hence, outside of the physical realm. As a result of being outside the physical realm, these subtle bodies that surround us cannot be seen in the physical sense. They exist on nonphysical planes of realty that can be seen intuitively or in a state of heightened awareness through meditation. Once you learn to enter a state of heightened consciousness, you will acquire heightened perception or awareness that allows you to see auras as energy fields that describe the condition of the subtle bodies that surround us.

In reading the aura bursts of energy, you will be able to determine what illness afflicts the totality of a living subject. We are more complex, you see, than what meets the eye in the physical self. That sort of physical observation simply skims the surface of our total being. In considering the wholeness of our being, we must consider maladies that afflict the emotional level of our being, the mental level of our being, and the spiritual level of our being for starters. These levels are not abstract, nor are they descriptive of inner qualities of our psyche. They exist as subtle bodies that surround the physical body like the outer layers of a bulging onion. They exist as halo extensions outside the physical body, representing the complexity of life beyond the simple physical explanation.

In truth, we are light beings. We radiate from the inside out. The rings of light that emanate from us reflect our true condition as plain as daylight. The colors and patterns of the light that radiates from us as glowing energy provide telling evidence about the condition of our chakra centers. To see all of this requires vision better than your eyes, as your physical eyes are limited to what is obvious only on the physical plane of existence. It requires a heightened sense of awareness that comes with the keen perception reached only in a state of heightened consciousness. This is the place frequented by natural healers who use their hands, heart, and higher mind to affect harmony and good.

Other animals know this place, too. So do plants. They walk close to nature. Consequently, they know the ways of spirit. Birds are psychic, as anyone can attest who has ever seen a flock all turn at once in the same direction or witnessed birds responded far in advance to a coming storm or other danger. Cats and dogs are psychic, too, speaking telepathically to each other and sensing things that are about to happen. And anyone who has lived closely with houseplants certainly recognizes that plants possess a heightened awareness in their natural ability to see around blind corners to find light and water to sustain them.

All of these living beings, like people, have energy fields that describe their condition of the many levels of their bodies including subtle bodies outside the physical self. In this sense, all of life is the same. We are complex, energy beings that live on many levels.

The light that radiates from our bodies is generated by chakras or *chi* centers that act as energy centers. The main energy centers in our bodies correspond roughly to the endocrine glands in the physical body. These chakras or energy centers exist on many levels and correspond to the many subtle bodies of our body, as well as our physical body. As the chakras emanate energy bursts from the body, beginning at the dense, core body that we call our innermost physical self, the energy assumes light colors that describe the filtering process that it goes through in leaving the body. The light colors of the aura, then, describe where the light has been and experienced.

It might help to think of the subtle bodies that our energy bursts travel through as filters. The subtle bodies filter out all color except one color that corresponds to a condition of that subtle body. If you know anything about light photography and its use of color filters, that's pretty much the way that camera filters work. A yellow camera filter tends to filter out pretty much all color except yellow. These filters eliminate colors other than the narrow range or light band of the color spectrum that it represents. This is the way all light reaches our world—through a prism effect that separates energy as light bands in a seven-color spectrum or scale.

The amazing thing about life is that the microcosm reflects the macrocosm. We reflect the way the greater universe works. As above, so below. That is because all of life is comprised of the same universal energy that is processed by all living things.

The colored lights that radiate from the living body, to the trained natural healer in a learned state of heightened consciousness, reflect the condition of the total being in its many levels of being. The colors of the aura describe the condition of the body, mind, and spirit. In learning to read and heal the chakras, the natural healer begins to interpret the tell-tale signs of illness as ragged energy fields and color bursts that immediately identify the condition of the being on many levels.

The natural healer learns that illness is basically energy anomalies that appear as energy shortage, blockage, or imbalance. Healing energy balance restores harmonic resonance to the living body, which is a self-regenerative organism capable of self healing with a little help from occasional energy boosts.

The energy healer works magically with nature to restore the harmonic balance within an ailing subject by restoring a proper balance of energy as needed.

Chapter 1

Many Applications

I'll never forget the beautiful, immense aura that I saw one Sunday afternoon in a community church. I must explain that I didn't frequent this place, but was attending to hear a particular discussion that was announced in the little weekly newspaper where I worked in that sleepy Oregon town. As a consequence, I found myself seated on a hard, wooden bench four rows from the front on the right side of the building. The view from this seat was simply dazzling. I saw a beautiful aura.

Well, every aura is unique, as I learned in time. Also, every aura is indicative of the person or life force that projects it. The aura, after all, is a personal manifestation of the energy that is most active in the host body at that particular instance. It changes from minute to minute, as personal focus and conditions change in the host body. In a real sense, people's auras are like colorful signatures of their precise identity, what they're really like, and how they really feel on many levels.

This particular aura in the church was astounding to behold. I remembering feeling a little guilty that not everybody in the room could see it, because it completely exposed the man who radiated this magnificent burst of dazzling light. It was his personal signature, open and readily apparent to anyone who could see it and distinguish the colors and patterns.

The aura might have belonged to anyone in the room. As it happened, it belonged to the clergy man who was standing at the head of the room behind a speaker's podium. He was very happy and enthusiastic; and it really showed. His immense aura radiated far above his head and on both sides of his shoulders in a gorgeous light show. There was blue light with sparkling gold highlights above it. There was pink light shooting out from him in all directions. There was green light, too. Best of all, the light was swirling in motion and dynamic, like the man who radiated it. Listening to the man speak, I could easily understand the light as a reflection of what was going on inside him. He was filled with love for the people that he addressed, exuding healthy good cheer for them and bubbling with a spiritual sense of sharing. I really didn't know this man, but gazing at his aura told everything vital about him at this particular moment in time. I remember thinking how lucky the people in that group were to have him as their friend and leader.

Unfortunately, most auras are not that beautiful, immense, or vibrant. Still, the color, size, contour, and liveliness of every aura tell volumes about the person who radiates this energy burst from the body. You might say that a person's true feelings spill out all over in tell-tale colors.

Most of the auras that I closely observed that summer in Oregon were darker, smaller, more ragged, and deader than the vibrant aura that I saw that one day in the church. That's because I was learning to consciously read auras of sick people in order to heal them by restoring life energy.

I hasten to add that there was nothing abnormally dark or sickly with our pretty, little mountain town. It's pretty much the same everywhere you look, when you read auras to diagnose and treat illness with energy bodywork. Eventually, you recognize certain signs about the way people feel by reading the color, shape, and vibrancy of their auras. This sort of aura reading can make a natural energy healer more effective, because the healer reads the person perfectly in colors that cannot lie. The aura is an accurate description of a person's immediate feelings and conditions that are most manifest energetically at that particular time. Anybody who can truly "see" in this psychic sense can read the signs. This is aura reading with a particular purpose and focus. Anybody can learn to do it and apply it with a little training, patience, and loving concern.

One of the local healers who taught me to read a person's aura for therapy was somebody I really trusted and respected for her work in a local hospice program. A nurse and founder of the hospice program had learned therapeutic touch healing from Dr. Dolores Krieger, author of *The Therapeutic Touch*. As a professor of nursing, Dr. Krieger has taught hundreds of thousands of nurses and healing professionals how to use their hands to help heal in a natural way through the transfer of body energy and energy all around us. Well, the woman from the local hospice program who taught me this healing technique combined it with aura reading.

As part of her personal training of me in energy healing, Karen had me scan people that we both saw walking across a public street. She did this at a slight distance, to avoid seeming intrusive. This was a real-life test to spot the sick ones and determine what needed to be done to assist with their possible healing.

We would stand at a street corner at a downtown intersection and just watch people. More precisely speaking, we *scanned* them. By that, I mean that we used a scanning technique to read and interpret their aura or colored light energy that radiated from their bodies.

Now you can scan many things psychically in this way by *gazing* at them. You can gaze into the clouds and interpret what you see. You can gaze into water and interpret what you see. You can even gaze into fire, candle drippings, or crystal balls. This isn't exactly the same as *looking into* something. More precisely, the person who gazes learns to look in a different manner, shifting the eyes a little to the left and staring with eyes a little out of normal focus. Then the gazer shifts into a heightened state of consciousness where perception is based more on heightened awareness than on physical senses. An impression of an image begins to take shape in this state. Then the higher mind sorts it out to interpret what is seen. This is psychic vision. It requires the third eye that is located in your forehead. Believe it or not, this really works. Centuries of psychic gazers and readers are proof of this. People pay good money for psychic readings.

Reading auras works about the same way as other forms of psychic gazing. The aura reader gazes with shifted eyes and slowly discerns an image. Generally, the aura reader sees a sort of white light like a soft halo around the head of the person who is being scanned in this manner. It helps, naturally, if the person who is being scanned for an aura reading is backlit by natural sunlight to accentuate the natural white halo of light around the head.

Once the aura reader has perceived the white light that surrounds the person who is being scanned, the aura reader begins to interpret the light around that person by tapping their higher awareness. The aura reader reaches a still, quiet spot deep inside himself, tapping the psychic insight of the third eye and higher awareness. The aura reader enters a meditative state of heightened consciousness to activate these internal functions. This is seeing beyond the range of your eyes. It is looking at light and discerning the colors of the light.

Professional photographers are well aware that light that we normally discern as white with our naked eyes has much coloration. The camera doesn't lie. Even bluish white light has at least six hues that the camera can detect. This is natural and not paranormal at all, when you think about it. Consider how light falls on everything on the earth, refracted in a prism effect into seven basic colors and their many subtle hues.

The seven basic colors of light, which are refracted in a prism effect upon entering the earth atmosphere, happen to be the same colors in the seven basic human chakras. For that matter, they are the same colors of the rainbow that you will find in the chakra system of a dog or a horse. Every body on the earth receives light energy and processes it in the same basic manner. And the light energy that every body receives has seven basic colors: Violet, indigo, blue, green, yellow, orange, and red. That is the color spectrum of color energy, as we receive it and process it within our bodies. And each color of light energy has properties and qualities that make it unique as light energy. Some of us naturally have more blue. Some of us naturally have more yellow.

These are the seven rays of light. They are literally gifts from the heavens that radiate down upon us in the form of heavenly sunshine. No living life form in our world could exist without these seven heavenly gifts. No living life form in our world could function dynamically without transforming this light energy and its many properties internally and externally. We literally consume and process this light energy within our bodies and project it outward as personal energy. Most of us are not aware how much energy we have and how beautiful it is. But all of us have it, or we wouldn't even be alive.

The ability to manifest and project this light energy outside of our bodies is something that can be practiced and perfected. I no longer consider this sorcery, although it is something that sorcerers surely do at will. Since I have worked with gifted healers like Karen and eventually Dr. Krieger, I recognized the inherent potential in all of us to direct this energy from our bodies for a good purpose, including healing others.

Moving energy and transformation with energy are definitions of magic, however. So I would have to say that the practice is truly magical. But it's magic that everyone does to a degree and can learn to do with greater perfection as a healing art form. Think of it as the art of living and the practice of giving.

Yes, every body processes light energy. And the light energy that radiates most unconsciously from your body is the energy that leaks from you as an overflow of the energy process that is most apparent within you. In short, the color of light energy that radiates from your body as your aura provides snapshot evidence of the energetic activity most prevalent in your body.

The colors of your aura can change from instant to instant, reflecting the different energy activity that dominates your internal processes. Moreover, the colors of your aura are filtered as they leave your body as a processing center for energy, passing through chakras and subtle bodies that serve almost like filters. So the colors of your chakra give a very definitive and detailed description of what is going on deep inside you on many levels. The colors that you radiate really reflect your inner being at that moment.

Reading the colors of people's auras on a street corner, as Karen taught me to do, became my exercise in spotting illness and transition in people. In some cases, it even showed me what impending death looked like. I learned to identify brown, black, green, and blue as typical auras colors regarding health and well being. Sick people that I scanned on the street corner often had brown in their auras. People in an advanced state of ill health often had grayish-brown auras or ultimately black auras. People who were sick, but beginning to heal, often had green auras or even bluish-green auras. There were subtle aspects to reading auras that I did not comprehend at that stage of learning to read auras. This comes with experience as an aura reader and as a natural healer. What I learned to read on the street corner with Karen as my teacher was simply how to spot fairly obvious and generalized aspects of aura coloration.

Actual follow-up to aura reading for health signs generally means energy body work. Or at least that is the way a natural healer would respond to definite health indicators in the people that they scan. My exercise in learning to read auras at a distance with special focus on health signs generally did not include follow-up healing sessions. That is because I was generally reading strangers as a learning exercise and did not have permission or even implied consent from any of these people to heal them. Permission for a natural healer is important. I could not simply send healing energy or approach any of these strangers.

My teacher, on the other hand, knew some of these people and had implied consent or previous permission from some of them to assist them as a healer. And she demonstrated to me that she could heal them even at a distance, unobtrusively. She impressed me with this ability on more than one instance.

"See that old man across the street?" she once asked me, looking intently in the direction of a slow-moving gentleman across the intersection that divided us from him.

I nodded, starring at him.

"Don't stare!" she warned. "Just watch."

I started to shift my eyes a little out of focus in the gazing technique that I had learned to be helpful in reading auras. Slowly I began to see the light around his head like a back-lit halo; and then I began to discern the subtle colors of the light. It was not colorful like most auras I had seen. Instead, it looked sort of dark like a soft, fading brown cloud around him. It was a small aura and not crisp. Also, there was a dirty mustard color swirled into it, as a sort of dark yellow undertone.

"He doesn't look good," I commented weakly to my friend.

"No, he's very sick," she said. "I know him. Now watch. I'm going to send him some healing energy."

She was quiet for an instant, as though focusing herself on her intent. It was as though she were gathering her healing energy to transmit.

"You can help, if you want," she said. "Just focus your attention on him and visualize sending him your best thoughts to get well. Then visualize your thoughts reaching him and actually making him well. You are sending him healing energy."

She stood transfixed on the street corner, directing her attention totally on that man across the way. Then she turned away and smiled.

"There," she said, beginning to walk down the street. I wanted some kind of explanation.

"That's it," she said.

I looked back at the man. He did look better. The brown aura around his head had given away to a little bit of green and blue. He looked a little more energized.

It took me some time learn that the actual healing was something that a sick person needs to do personally, not something a healer could bestow like a gift. The healing energy that the healer directs to the sick person only assists in this internal process, sort of like a stimulant or battery recharge for a weakened battery devoid of natural ability to regenerate.

But you can jump-start a car time and again without really restoring the full power to a car's energy reserves. Only when the vehicle recharges itself fully is it self-sufficient and healthy again. Sometimes a weak battery can be recharged by driving around carefully to recharge the battery. Sometimes the battery cannot recharge itself and will not accept a proper charge. So it is with people, who need to accept responsibility for healing themselves with a little help from their friends.

Healing, after all, is an internal process. A person who is sick ultimately heals himself or herself. What my friend Karen tried to teach me in reading auras of sick people on street corners was that auras describe our sickness in ways a natural healer can help. The way the healer helps is simply to send healing energy to assist in the natural healing process of rejuvenation. That healing energy can be in the form of healing thoughts, as in creative visualization, or even healing hands. There are many ways to send energy; and energy takes many forms.

Eventually, I saw a black aura on that street corner. It was the black cloud of death that everybody seems to dread; and it hovered over a good friend of mine. My friend saw me and met me on the street.

"What are you doing here—just standing on the street corner, watching people?" she asked.

I had known her for some time and knew her well, so I couldn't help but tell the full truth to her.

"I was reading auras," I told her. "Practicing my aura reading. You know that interests me. Well, that's what I was doing. You caught me!"

She looked at me with a cautious, sideways glance.

"Tell me, what does my aura look like? Right now," she said.

Her darkened eyes were foreboding and filled with apprehension. She looked so sad.

"Honestly?" I said. "Well, I see a sort of halo over your head. Only the color today is dark. I'm guessing that it's not a good day for you, because I don't see sparkly, bright colors. It looks sort of black."

"Figures," she said. "Like a black cloud over my head?"

I nodded, not knowing exactly what to say.

"I just learned that I'm very sick," she said. "Maybe that's it."

"Well, that's probably it," I said. "But black comes before all other colors. Everything comes out of darkness."

"Doesn't a black cloud mean death is coming?" she said.

It was one of those times when folk wisdom and metaphysical truth were pretty much the same. I couldn't deny that she was right.

"You know, it also means transition," I said. "Maybe it's a sign to get ready for a transition in your life—a time to put your life in order for the next phase."

She hugged me. Life, after all, is all about change and transformation.

That is true for all of us—people, pets, fish, flowers, and trees. Life is a process for all of us. As living creatures who absorb and process energy as colored light, we are all transformers. We transform ourselves and the world around us by the way we process energy. We utilize all seven basic colors of light in difficult ways for different purposes, realizing the unique and divine properties of each color of light.

The seven rays of light in the natural spectrum correspond to the seven colors that are associated with our chakras and our subtle or energy bodies. So you see, we are basically transformers of energy. We can transform energy in its many colorful forms to make changes in our life and the world around us. Consequently, our ability to bend and shape the colors of divine light within us and around us makes us agents of change. We can change ourselves and the world around us in many ways with the energy at our disposal, once we learn to channel it and direct it with focused intent and magical will.

Health or well-being can occur on many levels—physical, emotional, psychically, mentally, and spiritually. Using the energy within us and around us to establish health on many levels of our complex lives requires the full spectrum of the seven rays of light in our lives.

What I eventually learned by standing on that street corner with my friend as teacher was that everybody has all of the colors of the rainbow within them and the divine properties of the seven rays of light as transforming energy. How we use these seven rays of light determines how healthy and dynamic we are on many levels. Certainly, not all colors of light are equally active in all of us. Sometimes the very colors of light we need to activate within us lie dormant inside our bodies, waiting to be utilized.

Aura healing has many applications for both the healer and the individual who is concerned with the natural process of self-healing. I say that self-healing is a natural process, because individuals must ultimately heal themselves and can realistically expect to do this as self-regenerative dynamos of energy who can absorb, process, and transform energy to affect their own lives and lives around them.

The healer can use aura reading as a guide to determine the active, transformative process that is churning inside a subject's body and also determine what healing colors are lacking in a subject. Perhaps the healer can assist the subject by infusing the energy of the colors that are lacking. Or perhaps the best the healer can do is to assist the subject in stabilizing the internal process to reach a level of peace and tranquility.

Some people, after all, are terminally ill and cannot rejuvenate all the way back to perfect health. But they can find a comfort level. Some people need to work on issues that illness raises as a symptom of deeper concerns and must do this largely on their own, once they recognize the symptoms of their outward illness. Certainly not all illness is physical. Some illnesses are mental, psychological, and spiritual.

The practiced aura reader can detect illness by reading the color of energy that radiate from a body and also note which colors are absent. Recognition of the energetic condition of a body can aid both the healer and the subject in addressing what is happening deep inside someone. Then the healer and the subject can work to make adjustments in the energy field, often working together.

In a real sense, we are all terminally ill, because the physical aspects of our mortal coil will eventually decay and die. But we are more than physical bodies. The energy aspect of our life essence is non-physical and magical in the way it sustains us physically and energizes us. The energy that we absorb and process in this manner is eternal and cannot be destroyed. In that sense, there is a divine spark of the eternal within all of us, nourishing us day by day.

Chapter 2

Basic Aura Reading and Energy Scanning

The colors that radiate from our bodies as auras speak volumes about who we are and what we're all about. If you know what you are looking for, you can read the colors of the aura as a complete and detailed description of the person or other living thing that emits these colors. The colors basically describe the most active concerns of the person or creature that is generating the aura. The colors correspond to different energy in different phases of the body as a whole. Each energy wave or frequency corresponds to a color.

Everybody receives the full spectrum of colored light as a full complement of energy bands to process according to internal needs. But the colors that radiate or "leak" out of a person as an aura relate generally to the type of energy that is most active in the body at that particular time.

Of course, auras are subtle colors that are hard to detect without training. Anyone can learn to read aura, however. The easiest way for many people might be to position the subject in front of a window or otherwise backlight the subject so that natural light shines upon the subject's back as the subject faces you. Then you need to put yourself into a state of heightened consciousness with meditation to raise your awareness. The rest is simply the practice of gazing and psychic interpretation by reading the colors that you see radiating from the subject.

But before you attempt to read auras, it's most important to understand the meaning of the colors that you will see. There is some general consensus about the basic meaning of colors in mystic tradition, but certainly room for personal interpretation that involves psychic intuition. For this general discussion, however, we will reveal the traditional meaning attached to basic aura colors, based on the values generally given to these colors in occult studies and magic.

Please realize that each color has energetic properties that are unique to this color in the light spectrum. That is to say that each band of light has energy vibrations and characteristics that are unique to that color.

RED:

Red is often seen as the color associated with the root chakra or lower chakra (often called the first chakra). This chakra at the base of the spine governs the legs, feet, kidneys, spinal column, and stress responses, generally speaking. Also, it is associated with the adrenal gland, the psychological function of survival, and the will to live. In terms of illnesses, it is associated with anemia, blood diseases, circulation problems, constipation, paralysis, physical debility, and blood-related diseases.

Psychic healers generally regard red light as hot, vitalizing, and stimulating.

Red is at one extreme end of spectrum in a basic seven-color light spectrum, with violet at the other end of the spectrum. In terms of energy waves, the vibration of red as light energy corresponds to the sound frequency of Middle C in the diatonic music scale.

Many holistic therapists and musicians who work with music for healing recognize the qualities of sound to resonate with various chakras in the body, as they work toward a goal of harmonic resonance and balance. So they see how the middle C will correspond and resonate with the root chakra. All natural energy is pretty much the same, although we experience it in different ways. One way may be auditory, while another may be visual. Each color vibrates in its own way and can be associated with a musical note. In terms of sound, frequency is determined by how many sound waves are made in one second. In terms of light, color is determined by the number of light waves that reach the eye in one second.

As our bodies absorb and process red light, this particular band of energy brings with it special attributes that impact our lives in many ways. The color red is widely recognized metaphysically to stimulate sex, vigor, and overall strength. These are properties of the red light as energy.

Red in color therapy is also seen to act upon the urinary tract, rectal area, reproductive organs, and red blood cells. If we look at color as particular bands of light energy and think of energy as fuel for change, then it is easy to see how colors of light can act upon our bodies. Like all living beings that absorb and process energy, we utilize the light energy within us and use it to transform ourselves. In that sense, we are energetic dynamos or agents of change with the magical ability to transform energy.

Since we all have the magical and natural ability to transform energy, we can project light by visualizing that color band in our mind's eye and generating it. In a sense, color imagery is the internal ability to visualize color and the innate ability to recollect the vibratory feeling of that energy's signature pattern. Consequently, we can visualize color and send it outward to another person who might need the healing characteristics of that color of light energy.

Sometimes people unintentionally "spill over" with an overload of emotional feelings that they seem unable to contain inside them. People who "leak" red unintentionally may simply be experiencing a swelling of intensive, physical love. If you are attempting to heal a person by examining the aura and see such a color, you might note a smile and distant look on the face of such a person.

If you use red candles to stimulate and help heal the areas governed by the root chakra, remember also that the vibrational energy of red candles promote love, passion, and courage in a body. .

The color red is also associated with birth signs. Although not everyone agrees which colors match sun signs for the months of our birth, many people traditionally associate the color red with the birth signs Aries and Scorpio. People born under the sign Aries are born March 21-April 19. People born under the sign Scorpio are born October 23-November 21. Of course, the same holds true for dogs, cats, or even horses born at these times of the year. Their color is red. In a sense, it is their natural color. If you were attempting to heal them in a candle lighting ceremony, it would be appropriate to have a red candle present to represent their color essence. (This may be used in addition to a candle of another color and intent.)

ORANGE:

In color therapy, the color orange is often associated with the thyroid, kidneys, spleen, and colon. That is because it resonates with the second (sacral) chakra, which is located in the area of the abdomen. This chakra governs the reproductive system and lower abdomen and relates to the gonads, desire, pleasure, and the will to feel emotionally.

This orange color of light has other principles with regard to health. It is good to use on muscle spasms, such as spastic colon or colitis.

Orange light relates to asthma, bronchitis, epilepsy, nervous conditions, and mental disorders.

Psychic healers often view orange light as warm, stimulating, and vital to circulation.

Metaphysically speaking, orange is associated with stimulation, attraction, happiness, and kindness. It is even said that projecting orange light of a golden hue can bring fortune. Of course, fortune can mean different things to different people.

Musically speaking, orange light vibrates at the same frequency as the musical note D in the diatonic scale. A true master of magic, perhaps, could arrange the seven basic colors in a beautiful harmony that triggers the music of life. Certainly, it would be natural for anybody to process all of the colors of light in proper balance to restore whole body health and perfect harmonic resonance within the system.

Orange candles burned in a healing ceremony or as part of your aura healing session will act upon body areas governed by the second chakra and also act upon emotions and overall body energy.

Astrologically speaking, people born under the birth sign of Leo generally resonate to the color orange. They are people (or animals) born July 23-August 22. If you are attempting to perform aura healing on a Leo, you might be wise to project the color orange or work with an orange candle during candle healing to better relate to the energetic signature of the Leo.

YELLOW:

The color yellow has unique healing properties of its own. It is associated with the third chakra or solar plexus chakra that governs the stomach, liver, gall bladder, and upper abdomen. Yellow healing light aids our digestive system, liver, stomach, and lymph system.

This important chakra, as a swirling vortex of psychic energy, is associated with the pancreas, laughter, anger, power of the will, and mental will. Psychic healers generally see this chakra as soft, pastel yellow.

Yellow light energy, then, offers a positive magnetic vibration that has a healing effect on the nerves, as well as the pancreas and overall solar plexus region.

Physical sickness associated with malfunctioning third chakra in this region might take the form of constipation, diabetes, or even dyspepsia.

Another way to look at the characteristics of yellow light energy is musically. The vibrational frequency of this spectral band of light energy corresponds to the sound vibrational frequency of the musical note E in the diatonic music scale. Consequently, the playing of this musical note summons the same healing energy as yellow light in addressing the needs of the solar plexus region of the third chakra.

There are metaphysical attributes of the color yellow, as well, and these concern a body's overall psychological strength as seen in our mental and emotional power. Yellow light favorably impacts our confidence, comfort, persuasion, and intense thought.

You can use yellow candles in a healing ceremony or as an adjunct preparation to your healing session. Yellow candles promote mental powers, creativity, confidence, persuasion, and travel.

Yellow may also be considered a signature color for people (and other animals) born under the sign of Gemini (May 21-June 20), Virgo (August 23-September 22), and Pisces (February 19-March 20). True to the vibrational characteristics produced by their signature color, Geminis tend to be creative, confident, persuasive, and mentally intense. Virgos tend to be flexible, versatile, changeable, giving, and mission-driven. Pisces is changeable, versatile, flexible, and loving, as well. Energetic aspects of the color yellow help make Gemini's, Virgos, and Pisces people who they are. Yellow also suggests the kinds of health issues that each might have, as a positive or a negative. Yellow light is a gift with many benefits that are uniquely different from red or even blue colored light.

GREEN:

Green light energy corresponds to the fourth chakra or the heart chakra. This chakra governs the heart, circulatory system, arms, chest, and hands. It is also associated with the thymus and the qualities of loving, balance, and transformation.

In color therapy, green has proved effect in treating heart problems, lungs, thymus, and even headaches. Green light is also useful in healing as a vibration that stimulates balance and harmony with a soothing effect.

Metaphysical attributes of the color green include growth, wellness, fertility, finance, and energy. Green candles are often used to stimulate fertility, prosperity, and overall good health.

The energy of green light corresponds in terms of vibrational frequency to the wave sound of F in the diatonic musical scale. So playing the musical note F intensifies the energy of green used in healing. Even thinking about the musical note F creates this healing energy in the same way that visualizing green light inside your mind's eye creates such energy.

The birth sign Capricorn is associated with the color green. People born December 22-January 19 resonate with this color as their signature color. Capricorn people tend to be logical, keen, and accurate with solid determination to a life mission.

Green is considered an overall good healing color, because it stimulates growth and fertility. Green energy also helps the heart and lung. Your heart pumps the blood that flows through your body, carrying oxygen with it. It is a vital key to good health. Similarly, your lungs process oxygen that is essential to the body's good health.

BLUE:

Blue healing light corresponds to the fifth chakra or the throat chakra. This chakra governs the bronchial, vocal, lungs, ears, and respiratory system. Physically speaking, it is associated with the parathyroid and thyroid. Psychologically speaking, it is associated with grieving, communication, expressiveness, and higher emotions.

The color blue has been effectively used in color therapy for sore throat, laryngitis, hoarseness, palpitation, fevers, goiter, colic, jaundice, skin abrasion, burns, and cuts. Color therapists also use blue light to treat the larynx, thyroid, jaw, tonsils, mouth, and speech problems.

Psychic healers often see blue healing light as a cool vibration that relaxes, cleanses, and can even induce restfulness.

Blue light energy is soothing, calming, and protective. It can be used as an astringent. It can be projected to protect. Metaphysical attributes of blue light include serenity, sincerity, understanding, devotion, and truth.

Musically speaking, the energetic frequency of blue light corresponds to the sound frequency of the musical note G on the diatonic scale. So playing or projecting that note creates a focused amount of additional blue light energy to bring to bear to certain ailing parts of the body when needed.

Blue is also the signature color of people born under the sign of Sagittarius November 22-December 21. Sagittarius people (or other animals) tend to be charming, artists who are full of fire, adventure, and harmony. Blue is their signature color, and the magical properties of blue energy is their special gift.

INDIGO:

The color indigo relates to the sixth chakra, also known as the brow chakra in the area of the forehead. This chakra governs the eyes, nose, lower mind, and nervous system. It is also associated with the pituitary gland, medically speaking. Psychologically, it is associated with dreaming, imagination, visionary thinking, compassion, wisdom, and the personality.

We can use the healing rays of indigo light energy to treat hearing problems, eye problems, pneumonia, headaches, hormonal imbalance, developmental disorders, and even mental disorders. Eye problems addressed by indigo light energy include everything from inflammation to cataracts.

Indigo light works on the negative elements of the lower consciousness, as it relates to the lower mind in the general area of the forehead. It might help to think of indigo as magnetic, circular energy that takes hold and transforms.

Indigo is the color of people born under the sign of Taurus April 20-May 20. Their leading sense is hearing. Their characteristic magic is magnetic forces. They are adaptable to organization and enduring. Indigo is also the signature color of people born under the sign of Libra born September 23-October 22. They tend to be philosophical people who adapt well to organizations, and determine cause and effect. Like people born under the sign of Taurus, their characteristic magic is magnetic forces.

Metaphysical attributes of Indigo are transformation, ambition, and depression.

This is because indigo is linked energetically to the sixth chakra in the forehead, which is linked to our psychic self.

As pure energy, the wave frequency of indigo light corresponds perfectly with the sound frequency or vibration of the musical note A in the diatonic musical scale. Consequently, projecting this sound in your thoughts or out loud could amplify the healing effect of this energy's unique properties.

Purple candles also can be used to project the energetic properties of indigo light. In candle magic used for healing, purple candles are often used to develop the third eye, dream work, spirituality, and psychic power. Indigo light energy, after all, addresses the sixth chakra that governs this activity.

VIOLET:

Violet light acts upon the seventh chakra or crown chakra that is generally considered to reside slightly above the top of your physical head. This would be the same in other animals, of course.

The crown chakra governs the higher mind and is associated with the pineal gland. Consequently, it is the seat of higher knowledge, the soul, holism, and bliss.

Violet light energy can be directed to treat mental disorders, sleep disorders, and nervous conditions. Also, it will stimulate the higher mind, the soul, and spiritual bliss.

Metaphysical attributes of violet energy are power, piety, and melancholy.

A violet or purple candle can be used to stimulate the crown chakra and treat ailments associated with this chakra. Since it might prove difficult to find a violet colored candle, you might visualize indigo energy, as you burn a purple candle. Visual imagery can manifest energy and direct it, according to your will and intent.

The light vibrations of violet energy waves correspond to the sound vibrations of the musical note B in the diatonic musical scale. So you might project this musical sound in your thoughts or out loud in directing the divine healing properties of this particular energy.

People born with violet as their signature color are Cancer (June 21-July 22) and Aquarius (January 20-February 18). Not surprisingly, Aquarius people tend to be clairaudient, intellectual, light, elusive, and have a keen sense of smell. They are driven reformers. People born under the sign of Cancer tend to be clairaudients with a sharp sense of skill, as well. They are hands-on nurturers with a strong sense of will. Both are naturally nourished and blessed by violet light energy, as their bodies absorb and process this special energy.

SELECTING COLORS:

As we have seen, the full spectrum of colors present in refracted light is utilized by the body of people and other animals. Each one of us needs the full range of these healing color energies to process in our bodies and feed our chakras as internal energy vortexes.

Each color of light energy has unique properties and addresses particular areas of our bodies, as we transform energy within us. The above introduction to the seven basic colors of light energy serves as a guide to determining which colors to select in aura healing. Once you determine which colors are lacking in an aura and assess the weak chakra areas of the body, you can probably select the color of light energy that you want to project and direct in your healing efforts. Colors that are obviously present in the aura, on the other hand, will suggest to you what light energies are working in the subject, as they "leak out" or overflow from the subject.

In addition to an aura scan and assessment of energy deficiencies, however, the energy healer would be wise to practice a good measure of psychic insight in reading a subject for needs. This is a little bit like reading tarot cards, interpreting an astrology chart, or even gazing into fire, the sky, or a crystal ball. Psychic healing, after all, is divinatory in nature. Consequently, a natural healer who seeks to assess a subject's energy needs should always attempt to reach a state of heightened consciousness through meditation. Only in this state can the energy healer hope to have the intuitive ability that comes with heightened awareness.

Chapter 3
Our Subtle Bodies

As we have seen, our total being is much more than our dense, physical body. Our complete life essence includes a layered webbing of energy bodies that are invisible to the untrained eye. Hence, they are called *subtle bodies*, because they surround and encase the physical body. Traditionally they have been called everything from our luminous body to our spirit body, our light being, and our outer shell.

In attempting to read the aura and perform any kind of energy healing, it is important to learn to view our wholeness as much more than our obvious, physical attributes. Furthermore, it is helpful to the psychic healer to learn to distinguish or at least recognize the various subtle bodies that extend from our dense, physical core body. Each of these subtle bodies plays a part in our total being and represents a key aspect of our life essence.

Mystic healers generally agree that there are seven principle bodies present in all people, including our physical body. Together, they typically extend approximately 3-4 feet from our physical core. The bodies operate cooperatively as integral parts of the whole. Still, it is wrong to think of the subtle bodies as lesser appendages that simply complement the physical core body. Our seven principle chakras operate as swirling energy centers on all seven bodies. After all, these psychic energy vortexes operate on all levels of our being and require no physical housing. They are non-physical energy centers; and energy functions wherever it is needed and wherever it is called.

Consequently, the particular location of a certain color of light energy in the web of subtle bodies that surround us tells what sort of energy is active and abundant on that level of our being. Of course, the lack of a certain color on a certain subtle body tells what might be deficient in our wholeness at that time, as well.

To read the auric field that surrounds us, then, the serious aura healer should learn to distinguish the subtle bodies that surround us and the role that each of these bodies plays.

Our Seven Bodies:
- Physical body as inner core.
- Emotional body (closest to physical body)
- The mental body—rational thought (third layer outward)
- The causal body—insight (fourth layout outward)
- Individualized consciousness (fifth layer outward)
- Energized, conscious awareness (sixth layer outward)
- Divine essence (large, luminous outer shell)

Admittedly, many psychic healers and mystic seers disagree about the description of the seven bodies. Most generally agree, however, that humans and other living beings possess seven bodies including six subtle, luminous bodies that surround us like a web. The energy that surrounds us and impacts us on many non-physical levels of our being is simply not material or housed inside us. Obviously, our divine essence, conscious awareness, individualized consciousness, insight, mental powers, and emotions do not reside in our flesh, bones, or organs. They reside typically in our subtle energy bodies.

Often people refer to the subtle bodies that extend from our physical body as the auric field, because that is where the auras and their splendid colors are apparent, as they radiate from us.

Certain auras and the colors associated with them are associated with certain subtle bodies. The crown chakra and its signature violet energy is most obvious in the outermost seventh body, herein called our divine essence body. Indigo color of the brow chakra is generally most evident in the causal body layer of insightfulness. The yellow energy that drives the solar plexus chakra is most abundant generally in the mental body. Red energy drives the first chakra and is most apparent generally in the emotional body closest to the physical core. Blue energy, normally associated with the brow chakra, is often seen in the fifth and sixth bodies, which relate to individualized consciousness and energized conscious awareness, respectively. Nonetheless, we must begin to recognize that the chakra energy centers can operate and impact ALL subtle bodies that extend from us, as the colors of energy activity spill out into all aspects of our being.

It is easier for many aura readers, however, to recognize colors of energy that radiate from a person as associated with energy bodies where they are most obvious and commonly housed. This is because of a human failing, in part. All aura readers are physical creatures who are most familiar and comfortable when dealing with physicality and fixed physical locations. It is harder to recognize that colored energy moves freely within us and all around us.

At the same time, the aura reader who recognizes colors as meaning more than their assigned physical healing properties is correct in that reading. Blue energy sparkles that radiate far from the head, for instance, can indicate the expressive spiritual mindedness of a person or other animal (or even that of a tree, for that matter). At the same time, blue energy works upon our brown chakra, energizing our lower mind's expression. Green light is often seen as an overall good indicator that physical healing is taking place, although it is generally associated with the heart chakra. Red is often seen as love feelings that emanate from a person, although red is generally associated with the root chakra, reproductive functions and baser nature including anger. (Pink is also seen as animated love feelings that emanate from a person, like budding love of a gentle nature.)

None of these interpretations of the meaning of a certain color energy that surrounds the body is incorrect. These broader interpretations of color simply demonstrate the broad scope of these energies and the many properties that they bring to us as divine gifts of the seven rays. We tend to think primarily in terms of our physical nature and the comfort level of our physical bodies. We are much more, however, and so are the seven healing energies that impact our lives on many levels of being.

Since this book is primarily about healing, we will focus mainly on the colors of energy as they relate to the chakras in their roles in our physical body. At the same time, we will consider the emotional, mental, and psychic aspects of our overall health and well-being as spiritually whole persons.

Almost all healers around the world now have recognized the integration of body, mind, and spirit plus the way emotional well-being impacts us physically. In the same sense, spiritual depression impacts us both emotionally and physically. So we cannot ignore the interrelationship of the many levels of our being, as seen in the subtle bodies that surround our physical core.

In fact, the physical body may be the last part of us to realize the decay present in our subtle bodies. The physical ailments that we treat at the body level may first appear outside the body in the subtle bodies and gradually "fall to earth" to reside as symptoms in the dense, physical core of our being. Have you ever felt emotionally or spiritually troubled and then physically ill as a direct consequence? Everybody has. Many of the ills that bother us physically have their origins outside the physical body in the levels of our being that we call subtle bodies or spirit bodies. That would explain why allopathic medicine as practiced widely in the West is often ineffective in treating illness, since doctors commonly treat only symptoms of a condition that does not originate in the physical part of the body that eventually feels the pain. All parts of our total body from the cells in your toes to the crown chakra above your head are connected; and that includes your subtle bodies, as well. Tracing down ailments by treating places where you ache is a bit like tracing down electrical shorts in a vast network of buildings without schematic diagrams.

Sometimes an aching back suggests problems that simply treating the back can't cure. As author and healer Louise Hay has said, sometimes an aching back is a symptom of carrying too much baggage psychologically. Sometimes, then, symptoms are indicators that tells us something is wrong somewhere, even if the back looks strong and the overall physical body looks healthy.

We can ache in many ways. We can ache emotionally, mentally, psychologically, psychically, and spiritually. The three outermost levels of our subtle bodies relate to our spiritual awareness, awakened soul, and connection to the divine. Damage to our spiritual bodies will wound us on many levels, as the energy tears in these outer subtle bodies impacts the inner bodies and impairs our psychological state, mental well being, emotional state, and physical host body. We must always remember that the subtle bodies are connected. Damage to the outer shell of our being will eventually damage the inner core of our physicality and all layers of our well being. Think of a feather swirling in the wind, but then falling to earth when the wind stops. The orbit that keeps our subtle bodies energized and healthy is the chakra system that permeates our total being on all levels. A damaged chakra can happen in many ways, but is always crippling on many levels.

The Etheric Layer:

The subtle body that connects our physical body to our outer shells is the emotional body. An etheric layer is the innermost part of this emotional body and permeates both the physical body below it and the emotional body above it. In fact, many psychic healers consider the etheric body an almost separate subtle body by itself. It serves as a sort of connecting tissue. It also communicates between the physical body and the emotional body and outer subtle bodies. So the connection between our physical self and emotional self is very strong and immediate. Psychic healers who seek to energize the physical body often work with hands off the body to reach this important etheric layer.

The Emotional Body:

The emotional body that is so close to our physical core serves other important functions for us and other living creatures. It is the subtle body associated with our emotional energy. Admittedly, this is a different description of emotional energy from what most people are accustomed to hearing with regard to our base emotions and emotional outbursts. Our emotional energy is bio-magnetic energy that we channel from nature around us, process internally, and then project outward. We transform this energy within us and utilize it in unseen ways that most people do not consider. All of our psychic gifts are dependent on emotional energy that we transform within us. Like little dynamos, we process this energy and use it. Ultimately, healthy and well-rounded people who are functioning properly at this level can project it with will and intent. You don't need to be a psychic with lots of extra sensory perception from birth or special training to recognize this need. It's necessary for our instinct, foresight, sensitivity to danger and opportunity, and ability to read people and be read. We need a healthy emotional body to channel, process, transform, and transfer energy electromagnetically.

The Mental Body:

The second subtle body outward from our physical core is our mental body. This body is concerned with rational thought primarily. It is not our higher consciousness or insight, but our lower mind. Do not confuse the mind with the brain, which is part of our base physical body. The mind lives outside the physical body, with a natural connection to the physical body and the brain.

The mind is concerned with our mundane thoughts of a physical nature. It is concerned with the matters of the day and base needs and concerns related to the physical world. This is the lower mind's only reality. It does not operate outside the physical reality and mundane world of common, everyday matters. But mental breakdown of the mental plane of our existence can lead to mental disorders and irrational thought that impact our total existence including physical well-being.

The Causal Body:

The third subtle body, looking outward from the physical core, is the causal body. This plane of our existence is concerned with insight. In short, it allows you to truly know things deeply and intuitively, beyond simply knowing superficially about things. On the mental level, it is possible for the lower mind to know a little bit about a lot of things and relate to them rationally. This mental level activity, then, is a more superficial kind of knowledge than causal-level insight brings us. The causal body allows us to see beyond what our eyes can see and truly understand what we see. Of course, most people believe that they can read and study to attain insight. In truth, insight comes only on this plane of existence outside the physical body. Damage or decay of this important subtle body can impair your ability to have insight.

Many psychics also consider this fourth body to be the astral body that enables us to project our personality outside the physical body in astral projection and astral travel. Certainly, it is the highest level of subtle bodies of the three subtle bodies that are most closely connected to the physical self and the level where we deal with insight, causal connections, and intent. In a sense, it is our psychic body or psychic double.

The causal body, mental body, and emotional body are the innermost subtle bodies that are most closely connected to our physicality. That is true in terms of their proximity to the physical body, as well as their relationship to physical nature.

By contract, the outer three subtle bodies are more concerned with our spirit. They are concerned with higher consciousness, spiritual awareness, and our divine essence. Collectively, they form our higher self.

Individualized Consciousness:

The fifth body or fourth subtle body outward from our physical core houses our individualized consciousness. This is consciousness beyond our mental lower mind. This is consciousness of our higher mind that goes far beyond the limited, earthbound limitations of our physical brain or even our rational mind. It is the consciousness that we are actually individuals who can function on a very high level beyond the physical limitations of inward concerns for the bodily self. It is a heightened consciousness that identifies the individual with the cosmic consciousness and many levels of reality beyond the physical level. People who meditate to reach a higher level attempt to access this level. Like all subtle bodies or levels of our existence, this consciousness level must be energized properly and kept energetically healthy. It is our first connection with the spiritual world outside our base selves, as we attempt to reach outward.

Energized Conscious Awareness:

This is our sixth body or the fifth subtle body outward from our physical core. It goes beyond the range of individualized consciousness for the person who can energize and use this body. It reaches beyond the limitations of our physical perception with greater awareness that only comes with higher consciousness. And once that conscious awareness is energized, it can take you to distant places and exotic realities beyond the imagination of the physical self. This goes even beyond astral travel, as the range of the energized spirit body can take you to higher realms.

Divine Essence:

The outermost subtle body that extends broadly outward from our other subtle bodies is our divine essence or body that connects us to divinity. In some people who have realized their divine essence and worked in this subtle body, the energy field of this outer body is huge, extending many feet from the physical core. Typically, it extends about 3 or 4 feet from the physical core body, however. This is our divine connection or soul essence. Often this divine subtle body will radiate gold sparkles in a rich blue field in people whose spirituality is energized and becoming fully realized.

Luminous Egg Shells:

Seen together, the energized web of subtle bodies that surround our physical body make us look—to the psychic healer, at least, somewhat like a luminous egg shell. The subtle bodies wrap around us and radiate with energy. The many colors and properties of light energy that we absorb, process, and transform within us make us light bodies.

Or it might help to think of our layered light bodies as transparent, layered onion skins. Which layer of the onion is the actual onion? In truth, the many layers of transparent onion skins form the whole onion.

This book will primarily examine the health aspects of the body on physical, mental, and psychological levels. While we are concerned with spiritual well-being and growth, we are mainly focused here on how we become sick. As we have seen, we ache in many ways. What impacts us spiritually and psychically can affect us also deep within our inner, physical core. Just as emotional and mental level problems can make us physically sick, spiritual level problems can make us ache physically and impact every level of our subtle bodies.

So we cannot overlook the connection of all aspects of our being in considering what makes us ill. The auric energy field that surrounds us is a total package and must be viewed and treated as part of our total being.

Nonetheless, most of our immediate concern in reading auras in our energy fields will be focused on the physical body and to some degree the emotional, mental, and causal body that are closest to our physical core. We see the colored light energies of these subtle bodies most interrelating with the physical body that is so near and dear to them.

We will learn to read the auric energy fields that surround our physical bodies and the bodies of other animals with special regard to health, healing, and well-being to determine what energy is present and what energy is lacking. This involves seeing with more than our physical eyes, but seeing with new eyes of intuition and divination.

As energy healers, we will learn how to interpret what we have seen in aura reading and respond accordingly. We will project energy of precisely the right colors of light that correspond with the stressed chakras in question. These healing light energies of various colors will have the precise properties that are required to stimulate our friends in need and assist them in their self-regenerative effort. For some of us who are auditory by nature, we will also learn to project various healing sounds that correspond to the stressed chakras in the same way that healing color light stimulates them.

Chapter 4

Spotting Illness in Our Aura Energy Field

It is not easy to spot illness in the auric energy field, but always rewarding when you can identify it and interpret what you have read to begin healing treatment. Often the aura will be hard to read—at least at first, and difficult to distinguish on any sort of common color chart. The colors at first might appear to you as different intensities of white light. Even when you learn to read the colors, they tend to run together in a sort of swirl of colored light energy that is leaking from the body. Most people, it must be admitted, have not consciously learned how to transform color within them and have not learned how to project color. So color just leaks out of most of us, while we seem to try to hold it back, almost self-consciously.

Our first consideration in the task ahead is to realize how reading the aura is vastly different from normal seeing. Reading to a psychic healer means seeing with more than physical eyes. It is seeing with your total awareness. It is a form of divination in which the seer looks beyond the physical plane and the veils that surround it. The seer engages psychic intuition and perceptive awareness to replace the mundane physical senses. So do not expect to open your eyes wide and see colors swirling about. Really, you must learn to open your third eye. That is your eye of extra-sensory perception and divination. Everybody has this third eye, but must learn to acknowledge it, trust it, and use it.

Case Study Profile:

Professionals and efficient amateurs also want to compile a brief profile of the subject prior to treatment, which therapists often call a patient profile. This can be done on a single sheet of paper very simply. This is your opportunity as an aura reader and chakra healer to obtain clues about what is wrong with your friend, based on overall history, previous health conditions, symptoms, and other pertinent things that might induce physical, emotional, mental, and psychological trauma. In short, what seems to be troubling your friend? We want to get down to what seems to be malfunctioning in your friend's self-regenerative system. Consequently, we will ask a few questions or ask the friend to jot down responses to formatted questions in writing. This shouldn't be intrusive, but rather helpful in determining which chakras are not producing enough energy to sustain health, based on what parts of the body might be ailing. You might need to review Chapter 2 to match body areas with chakras.

You might include the following questions:

CHAKRA READING & COLOR HEALING

SUBJECT QUESTIONNAIRE

Name:_____ Date of Birth:_____

List any health problems you have had:

_____
_____
_____
_____

List any current health problems:

_____
_____

List any symptoms you have noticed:

_____
_____

Are you being treated for any condition? (Include medication):

_____
_____

List any stressful situation that might conceivably impact your health:

_____
_____

Comments:

_____

_____

_____

NOTE: This information is strictly voluntary and confidential. Chakra healing is not medical diagnosis or medical treatment, but only a supplement to proper medical care. You are encouraged to seek professional medical care for any health issues.

Setting the Stage:

It might help you to set the stage to read the aura of your ailing friend. Try putting your subject on a straight-back chair with the sun to your friend's back. This can be done outdoors or inside in front of a window. The idea is that the backlighting makes it easier to see light bouncing off your friend.

Ideally, your friend will be prepared for the aura reading and healing session. You should ask your friend to remove shoes, sit erect and firmly grounded with both feet anchored, and enter a meditative state. Now, this isn't entirely necessary, but helpful. Grounding and centering people in this manner focuses them on internal concerns and ensures that they aren't preoccupied with external matters. Once your friend is grounded and beginning to center quietly, you might intone a few words to help the friend focus on the matter at hand. For instance, you might say that you want your friend to silence the internal and external chatter around him (or her) and then find that quiet, still spot deep inside. Then you might suggest to your friend to focus on the healing process and get in touch with his (or her) total being.

To get your friend into a meditative state, direct your friend to plant both shoeless feet squarely on the ground and assume a rigid posture with a straight back. Do this softly and gently in a sort of monotone voice to guide your friend into deep body sleep that is similar to a hypnotic state. Suggest that your friend's body is going to sleep, beginning with the feet that grow heavy and then numb and followed by the torso, arms, hands, fingers, upper body, and head. Tell your friend that this numbness is normal and something your friend should allow happen. Tell your friend that the mind will stay awake, as the rest of the body falls into deep and restful sleep. Then suggest to your friend to clear the mind of all internal and external distractions, forgetting the concerns of the day and the endless mind-loop of concerns about yesterday and tomorrow. Then ask your friend to tune out all external distractions, so that the physical senses are numbed. Suggest that your friend simply focus on what you are doing for him and the healing process at hand.

You might also suggest that you want an accurate picture of the kind of energy and health issues at work in the total body at that time and will be reading and scanning your friend to help him. Assure your friend that you are going to help in the self-healing process, by touching your friend's energy with your energy and the natural energy around you. You should do this is a quiet, monotone voice that helps put your friend into a comfortable meditative state. After speaking these few words, become very quiet yourself.

Preparing Yourself:

You should prepare yourself in much the same way. Take a few seconds after positioning your friend to ground and center yourself, putting yourself into a state of heightened consciousness with heightened awareness. If you are unpracticed or find it difficult to enter this state, make your personal preparations before orienting your subject. Otherwise, put yourself into a heightened state immediately after orienting your subject.

You will not remain grounded in the same way that your subject is grounded with feet anchored squarely on the ground. You might start this way, but will find it necessary to move around during the healing session.

You will need to enter a state of rapid beta brain activity in active meditation. Pranic healers who work with energy might need to move around and keep acutely alert during healing sessions. So your meditative state will be more active, as opposed to the more passive meditative state of your healing subject. You will enter a state of heightened awareness where your eyes are slightly out of focus and your spirit guides you. You are straddling the line between the physical world and the world of spirit in this state.

Reading the Colors:

At first, you might see only white light that radiates from the head and shoulders of your friend in front of you. You are seeing only with your eyes at this point. You must shift your eyes a little out of focus and gain new focus with your third eye of psychic insight. Take the light in, and then see how it feels to you on a spirit level of perceptive awareness. Little by little, you will begin to sense the colors and properties of the light energy around the head and shoulders of your friend in front of you. Do not hurry the process. Give yourself time to interpret the colors deep inside you. This is not superficial light reading. Most people see light simply as it bounces off objects indirectly and then absorb it superficially with their eyes. At the light reaches ours eyes indirectly, the eyes take in the light much like a camera lens. And like a camera lens, we see upside down and then attempt to right the image internally. So we never see light or the colors of light directly, nor do we see with deeper clarity. We are like instant cameras that take quick, fleeting snapshots of what we think we see and then attempt to give it some meaning, based on our previously arranged frame of reference.

Interpreting Light Colors:

Interpreting light colors that radiate from the auric energy field of friends and other life forms that we hope to help heal energetically is the key to aura healing. This is not easy at first, because the colors of light energy are soft and exotic. They swirl, blend, and change before us. We must take it all in with new eyes of awareness. Consequently, it's important for the aura reader to remain in a state of heightened consciousness with eyes shifted, calmly waiting for the colors to reveal themselves to us.

We are looking for soft yellows, faded blues, exotic greens, unusual reds, swirls of purple, and pastel hues that rarely find themselves in our color photographs or on the canvas of any painting masters. These are the healing energies of light from the divine seven rays that rain down from the heavens and enter our bodies for processing and transformation with us. They energize us and make us whole, enabling our bodies to function on many minute levels. We need a full range of energy to thrive. Everyone needs the entire supplement, as every color of light energy has unique properties and function. People and other living creatures that are ill on any of a number of levels are deficient in some of these light energies.

Allopathic medicine often laments that it does not exactly know what makes our bodies move and function, acknowledging only the physical system of skeletal structure and system of pulleys and impulses that mechanically work within us. But our body is much more than a system of mechanical levers, switches, and superstructure. It processes and transforms energy, as seen in our neurological system and bioelectric system of infinite wonder.

We are looking not just for colors that are present or absent in the aura, but also anomalies in the energy field that surrounds our physical body. Rarely is an aura uniform, full, and rounded with solid color patterns. Often there are breaks, tears, ragged sections, swirls, and protrusions. That's true of the unhealthy life form; and many people are unhealthy to some degree.

Rest assured that nothing you do in reading the aura, interpreting the aura, or projecting healing energy to stimulate a person's self-rejuvenation can harm them. You are simply attempting to "jump start" that person's own batteries. The real healing is done by the ailing people who process and transform healing energy within themselves. The real healing is always done by the sick person, as any honest healer or medical doctor will tell you. We are all self-regenerative dynamos who process and transform energy internally. As an aura reader and chakra healer, the best thing that you can do is to stimulate the self-healing process by directing energy into the ailing person to absorb and process.

This is very evident in Kirlian photography, where an outside energy "burst" impacts a subject that responds to the outside stimulus with its own radiation discharge, seen on the Kirlian film as a corona discharge that resembles an aura pattern of energy emanating from the subject.

So the first task for chakra healers is to read the aura of the sick person or animal in front of them to interpret what color of light energy is lacking in the subject, since each color of light has different healing properties within the body.

Scanning with Hands:

To determine where there might be energy blocks in the body, it might be helpful to scan the body with healing hands. This can be done gently and unobtrusively with hands a few inches off the body. In this mode, it is critical that the chakra healer remain in a state of heightened awareness and totally focused on the task at hand. Your hands will give you clues. You can start above the head and work your way slowly down the body to the feet, being careful not to actually touch the person physically. You are reading the auric energy field that surrounds the body.

As you assess the body with your hands, you should become sensitive to any tingling in your hands, heat in the hands, or coldness in you hands. Or perhaps you will sense a hollow feeling or emptiness. In this application of pranic healing, you are using Psychometry or the divination art form of sensitive hands to guide you. Think of your hands as a double helix to send and receive energy signals or impulses. In this method of assessing the body, your hands are in a receiving mode and sensitive to the energy signals pulsing from the subject body in front of you.

You must get a working "feeling" for what the signals mean to you. Energy blockages take many forms, but always suggest a lack of healthy flow within the body. Perhaps there is an energy overload in one part of the body or else an energy shortage. Think of how a river becomes blocked in ways the waters remain in one place and do not flow to another place downstream. Our bodies are much the same. Energy flows through our body, but not always evenly in a healthy fashion. Where are the breaks, gaps, or blockages of energy in the body? What colors are associated with the health and well being of that part of the body? It might help to familiarize with the color correspondences in Chapter 2, so you know what colors of energy are associated with certain parts of the body that you are scanning. When you scan the body in this fashion, you find clues that can be associated with certain color deficiencies in terms of energy that is not flowing properly somewhere in the body.

One way to assess the body's energy in this manner is to start from a standing position directly behind your seated subject. You might hold your hands fanned out high over your subject's head. Your hands should be partially cupped to conform to the shape of the head, with your thumbs touching or nearly touching. While you generally want to avoid talking, particularly avoiding small talk, you might want to pose a question to your subject to orient both of you to the process. You could ask your friend to tell you when your friend senses something on or about the head. Then slowly begin lowering your hands toward the top of the head. Normally people will sense the energy from your hands meeting their own energy field above the crown chakra about a foot or two above the head. Then you can ask your friend to tell you when the sensation becomes very acute, beginning the process again. Most energy healers will feel heat, pressure, or an energy build-up of some kind, as their hands approach the emotional body and the etheric plane that is just an inch or two above the physical body. You might linger in that position just an inch or two above the head, so that both you and your healing subject become familiar with the sensation of your energies blending.

Of course, it's critical that you remain in a heightened state of consciousness, an almost trance-like state where your mind is racing, your body is somewhat numbed, and your focus is very fixed on the healing process. Your spirit body is extremely alert and reading energy signals.

Once you have made contact on a spirit-to-spirit level, spread your hands wider and facing each other and begin moving your hands down the sides of your subject's head very slowly, being careful not to make physical contact. (If you make physical contact, different senses come into play, destroying the perceptive awareness that you have been using in place of your five physical senses.) Avoid moving around much. This could disturb your subject and could disturb your own heightened state of conscious awareness. You are scanning the body now for anomalies in the uniform energy flow within your subject's physical body and etheric level. You could sense these anomalies as a warm spot, cold spot, empty feeling, tingling, or congestion. Be open to any and all sensations to your hand, as interpreted by your conscious awareness in this state. You might ask your friend to tell you if your friend senses anything warm, cold, tingling, congested, or hollow. Do this with as few words as possible, using a soft, monotone voice that will guide the subject in a meditative state without jarring your subject back to normal, physical consciousness. Both of you need to remain quietly focused and centered in a state of heightened consciousness.

Kneeling as you work your hands down your friend's back, slowly continue to move your hands downward on both sides of the torso, pausing wherever you might sense some energy anomaly or receive feedback from your friend, who sense any anomaly. Keep your hands facing each other from each side of the subject's body.

If you do not have any sensation whatsoever in your hands, then you might need to rise to your feet and refocus yourself. During body scans of this sort, you should sense some slight warmth or tingling in your hands that is not usual in your normal physical consciousness. If you do not feel this in your hands or sense it, then you should quickly rise to your feet and consciously center yourself to put yourself in this heightened state of consciousness. You might even rub your hands together gently to introduce the role of double helix feelers to your hands. Your hands should be operating together magnetically with a sensitivity to their shared role.

When you have completed the scan from the backside and scanned the body thoroughly to include the bottom of the spine, then you should quietly move to the front of our subject. Most likely your subject's eyes are closed in a meditative state, but it matters not either way. Do not make eye contact. Simply begin the body scan for energy anomalies from the front side, with your hands facing inward toward each other from either side of the head. Keep your hands a couple of inches off the body at all times. Focus on the feeling of your hands facing each other, with the subject's body between them. Do not project any energy at any time during this assessment scan, but focus only on receiving information from the subject's own energy field.

Moving your hands slowly down the front body of your friend, pause wherever you sense any anomaly. Determine what chakra area governs that part of the body and what healing colors are associated with that part of the body. You might quietly ask your subject for confirmation if you sense any anomaly without leading your friend to any conclusion. You might simply ask if they feel anything different at that point. Your friend should not need to physical look where your hands are located at that juncture, but sense where your hands are making contact with their body at that point. Do not discuss the sensation at length, however, but just seek confirming feedback.

Also scan the arms and hands, as you face your friend.

When you reach the torso of your seated friend, you may need to kneel in front of your friend to finish scanning the lower half of your friend's body. Do this as effortlessly as possible. You need to remain in a state of heightened consciousness and avoid getting too physical, or you may find your consciousness back in your physicality. You don't want to get back into your body just yet.

Complete your energy scan down your subject's legs, including the feet. Do not ask your subject to lift feet or move any part of the body, however. Your subject should remain grounded and centered without body movement.

It's often wise to do the full body scan from the back and also the front twice or more, as required. Often the initial scan will not produce enough information. Sometimes the healer is not sensitive to the information, but requires exposure to become sensitized to the subject's own energy field. Also, the signals might be subtle or even masked.

In scanning the body a second time, the healer can begin from the feet and work upward to avoid excessive movement. Admittedly, some healers who do body scans have the opinion that the energy should not be ruffled one way or the other in working either downward or upward on a friend. In this mode of assessing energy levels in the body, however, the healer is only receiving energy signals and not sending energy into the subject's body. Therefore, there should be no difference in working down the body or up the body. You may discover your own attitude toward this with practice and determine what feels right to you. Trust your instincts in this state of heightened awareness. Learn to read yourself, as well as your subject, as you scan in this manner.

Remember that this sort of body energy scan can be done with any living being. You can do it with you dog, cat, or horse in the same way that you do it with a person, basically. Naturally, pets will not always remain as quiet and still. It is surprising, however, just how still and quiet pets will become during such energy work. That's particularly true of dogs and horses. Cats often are a bit more fidgety. You might attempt to place a pet into a grounded space. Naturally, they might choose to sit or stand. Calm them physically by petting them gentling and talking to them in a quiet, soothing voice at first. Even though they cannot speak to you, unless you have a telepathic bond with your pets, expect them to offer feedback in body language. Often a pet will present to you a body part that needs attention by protruding that part of the body and putting it squarely in front of you for consideration. This, also, can be a significant clue in determining energy anomalies.

Once you have completed your body energy scan, return to a position facing your subject. It might be good to ground yourself in a chair in front of your subject. Return to reading you subject's aura from a distance by gazing with shifted eyes. You do not physically see with your eyes to any degree in this manner, but only use your shifted physical focus as a sort of guide or compass. You need to practice non-physical seeing in the way a seer gazes and makes a reading. You must see with your third eye of intuition and insight that is only activated in a state of heightened awareness. So you remain in an active meditative state, with your physical body still basically numbed. It is the spirit side of you that does all of the real work here.

As you gaze at your friend in front of you to read your friend's aura, what colors of light energy do you see? Be patient in making your reading. If you see only white light at first, do not despair. You are seeing the energy field that surrounds your friend. You simply need to focus on interpreting the actual colors of this light. The colors are subtle, swirling, blending, and changing. They tend to be soft, pastel hues. They are extremely faint and hard to distinguish at first.

If you find it impossible to see even a white light halo around your friend's head and shoulders, then you might move to more natural sunlight outdoors or near a bright window where the sunlight strikes your friend's body from the back in a backlit effect. This makes it easier to see the light around your friend, radiating off your friend's head and shoulders. It is not impossible to read auras in other light conditions including indoor situations with only artificial, interior light. It is simply harder in these unnatural conditions without strong, natural lighting that backlights your subject. Think of it as natural framing.

As you patiently gaze at your friend's health aura, subtle colors that surround the physical body should become slowly apparent to you on a deep, intuitive level. What appears first as white light radiating off your friend's head and shoulders gradually assumes pastel colors in your mind's eye. Typically, you see yellows, greens, blues, and reds in an aura. Occasionally, you see purples and orange. Based on the healing properties of different colors we have examined in Chapter 2, you should be able to determine what healing colors are active in a person. If you see green, for instance, it suggests that your friend is actively healing and projecting much green light energy. This could relate to the heart. A careful case profile and body energy scan should give you clues what areas of the body have energy problems. If the colors of the chakras that govern these areas are not present in the health aura, then you might conclude that your friend's self-regenerative system is not absorbing and processing enough of those particular colors of energy.

Of course, colors have other meanings outside physical, emotional, and mental health, as we have seen. Pinks oozing from a person's aura could mean love feelings, for instance. We are basically concerned with treating physical illness and looking for the colors that relate to the chakras in terms of physical health..

Other colors that might be apparent in a sick friend are gray and black. We have not discussed them, because they do not relate to any of the chakras that govern parts of bodies. Nonetheless, they are indicative in a health aura of a person's overall health condition and should be noted. Gray generally suggests a grave illness and reason for concern. Consequently, gray in a person's aura would encourage you to begin chakra healing immediately. Black in a person's health aura generally suggests death hanging over this person. Upon seeing black in a person's health aura, you might consider counseling this person about life transition. You needn't mention death, but only the major transitions in a person's existence as an energetic life force. Death is only transition in the broader scope of things, when you consider that energy never dies. As energetic beings, therefore, we may never die. Energy cannot die, but only changes. Change is transition. And transition is a part of living. We cannot even consider black anything necessarily gloomy and hopeless. Out of blackness, all things come. Out of the dark void comes new life. And in another sense, death is the ultimate cure for impossible health conditions.

Most people that you might treat as an aura reader and chakra healer will make their colorful energy apparent to you in ways that you can read and interpret, once you know a little about their condition and also know the color correspondences of the chakras.

Chapter 5

Preparing for Energy Healing

Both the chakra healer and healing subject should make special preparations for this kind of energy work. Energy healing, after all, is a special rapport between two beings and must be entered with the greatest reverence and respect for each other. In exchanging our energy with another in an attempt to help that person heal, we share the very essence of our being. We share our luminous being, our light being, our spirit. So we connect during energy healing spirit to spirit, becoming closer and more interconnected than most people could imagine possible. But when you think about it, all of life is interconnected. We share the same oxygen, water, energy, and images in a shared environment. We are all children of nature, which nourishes us with its life-regenerating light energy of the seven rays. As light from the sun enters our earth atmosphere, it is refracted by the prism effect of the earth's atmosphere curvature that bends the light into a radiant spectrum of seven colors. Each of these colors has a different frequency or vibrational intensity that can be scientifically measured. Consequently, each color of light has distinctive properties. This rainbow of natural life energy rains down upon all of nature's children and empowers us. We absorb this pure light energy in its subtle colors and absorb it, process it, and transform it inside us. We are all sustained and regenerated by the same universal energy. Since this energy is universal and nurturing to all life forms, we can share this energy to those whose personal energy supply is critically low. We know when a person's energy supply is low, because they become ill physically or on other subtle levels. Because all living beings in nature absorb, process, and transform this universal energy for self-regeneration, we can share our energy with other animals and even plant life as aura healers. We stimulate and relate to them in basically the same way that we share energy to help human friends in need—spirit to spirit.

This universal energy that we can magically transform within us and all around us is a gift of spirit on a grander scale, as it rains down upon us freely from the heavens above our mortal plane as gifts freely given. And so we want to return this gift and repay Spirit by sharing this divine blessing. Now many people, it is true, go through life with their hands clenched most of the time, unwilling to share. We live with many competitive people who have not learned the blessing of giving. In a sense, they have not realized the blessing of sharing. Perhaps they are too concerned about opening up and possibly losing something. In that closed-down position, however, they also are not open to receiving; and that's a sad thing, indeed. They have not become what some psychologists and mystics call self-realized. They have not realized their broader connection and the cosmic connection that binds us all together. They are not dead, but not totally alive, either. They are sleep-walking through the dynamic process of growth and change that we call living, not fully conscious.

Consciousness is a much broader concept than they can realize. Because they are functioning on a physical level, enjoying basic creature comforts, they assume that they are awake and alive. Actually, they are only functioning in a lower state of consciousness, the basic feeling of their bodies. Consequently, they live only superficially in their physical bodies, not really in touch with their higher mental bodies, emotional bodies, or spirit bodies. This is sad, but we can even reach out and stimulate these base creatures who share our world by sharing energy with them and communing on a spirit-to-spirit level. For them, of course, the experience of chakra healing will become an awakening.

Length of the Session:

An entire aura healing session could last as long as 45-60 minutes, but should not be any longer. The session should include three basic parts: (1) Orientation and Profile, (2) Energy Scan and Assessment, and (3) Energy Healing. Each portion will last approximately 15-20 minutes, but can be shorter. In particular, the energy scan and healing segments should not exceed 15-20 minutes each. Touching a person's energy body during scans and energy healing can prove exhausting to both parties.

Orientation:

As aura readers and energy healers, we start the session by orienting the ailing subject to the process and procedure. We tell our sick friend about the process step by step and prepare our friend to the friend's role in the process. You should tell your friend that you will be scanning his or her aura to determine what type of energy appears active and what type of energy appears needed at this particular time. You might tell your friend that you will do a visual aura reading to observe the color of energy around the head and shoulders area and may also perform an energy body scan. Assure your friend that you do not need to make tactile contact in order to do this. In fact, you will not be intrusive in any way. This should be comforting. Simply ask your friend to tell you if anything during the session makes your friend feel uncomfortable. You should respect this and even end the session, if your friend requests you to do so. It is not very likely, however, that your healing subject will experience any sort of discomfort or want to end the session, since the healing session should be very relaxing and rejuvenating. Most people remark that they feel much better at the end of a session, due probably to the relaxing nature of the meditation involved and the energizing aspect that leaves the healing subject feeling stronger and livelier.

In addition to the patient questionnaire listed in Chapter 4, the energy healer should maintain a case file with a record of all patient sessions. This should be updated with each healing session, incorporating information from the patient profile. It might look something like this:

CASE FILE

Name:_____ Date of Birth: _____

History of Chakra Healing Sessions

_____
_____
_____
_____

Describe Current Health Condition:

_____
_____
_____
_____

Under Current Treatment or Medication? (List):

_____
_____

What are the symptoms?

_____
_____

List any stressful conditions that might possible affect patient health:

_____
_____

How would you assess patient energy level at this time?

_____
_____

What, if anything, do you suspect might be wrong?

_____
_____

NOTE: This information should remain strictly confidential and is optional. The energy treatment that your healing subjects receive is not intended to replace medical attention, which is strongly recommended to diagnose and treat any serious health problem. This energy treatment is totally safe and harmless and intended only as a supplement for professional medical treatment.

Orientation is also necessary for the aura healer and a useful opportunity to gather information from the healing subject. You should ask your ailing friend to tell you pertinent medical history or any symptoms, assuring your friend that this information will be held in strictest confidence. Where does your friend sense pain or problems? What does your friend think it might be? You might develop a little case study intake chart to collect this sort of information from your ailing friend who can fill out the form much the way therapists and medical professions collect patient profile information. It's always advisable to tell your friend, too, that this energy healing is not a substitute for professional medical examination and treatment, which is also recommended. Nothing in energy healing is dangerous or counterproductive to professional medical care, but can supplement medical care.

It's important to tell your ailing friend exactly what he or she should do during the healing session. In a sense, you will do all the work, with your friend just sitting there quietly. Actually, the healing subject needs to ground, focus, and enter a meditative state for best results.

Now ask your subject to sit very erect in a straight-back chair with both feet firmly anchored on the ground—ideally with shoes removed. Then ask your subject in a soft, monotone voice to become very still and quiet, tuning out all external and internal distractions. Ask your subject to only hear your voice and focus only on your voice and the healing process. All other internal thought or observations should cease at this point, as your subject attempts to ground and center with focused intent. You might ask your subject to find a personal still point deep inside where everything is quiet and peaceful and then clear the mind. At this point, you could ask your friend to begin feeling feet and legs grow heavy and go to sleep, followed by torso, arms, chest, neck, and head. Tell your friend that the body is going into a deep sleep, but will remain safe. Meanwhile, assure your friend that the mind remains very much awake, focused totally on the healing process and nothing else.

Next, you will want to softly tell your friend that you will be observing your friend's aura to observe the different properties of energy at work. Say that you will do this visually by looking at your friend's aura and then, perhaps, by performing a body scan with your hands to the side of your friend's body. Make certain that you assure your friend that you will not be actually touching the body at any time, but will keep your hands a few inches off the body to assess any possible anomalies in the body's energy field. Your friend could be helpful in giving you some feedback when you do a body energy scan; and you should ask your friend to tell you about any sensation of warmth, tingling, coldness, or emptiness during this time, keeping conversation to a bare minimum.

Tell your friend that he needs to remain in a very quiet, centered state of heightened consciousness and remain focused on the healing process and nothing else, except for your voice.

Background tools:

You might also have colored candles, colored lights, and even sound to supplement the energy healing. It would be wise to bring the colors of candles or colored light that correspond to the seven healing colors that are associated with healthy chakras: red, orange, yellow, green, blue, indigo, and violet (Chakras 1-7 from root chakra to crown chakra, respectively). Once you have assessed which color of light energy is needed to revitalize your ailing friend, based on which chakra area is weakened, you can use the corresponding color to help project that color of light to stimulate the self-regenerative system in your friend's weakened chakra. The use of sound works the same way, since sound wave frequency corresponds to light wave frequency, if you know the correspondences. It's simple, really. Red corresponds to Middle C. Orange corresponds to D. Yellow corresponds to E. Green Corresponds to F. Blue corresponds to G. Indigo corresponds to A. Violet corresponds to B. Remember that energy can take many forms. Sound energy equates to light energy. You can play the note on a bell, piano, or guitar to resonate with the chakra that corresponds to that note and that color of energy. This is the approach of harmonic resonance and can be used to supplement your energy work. You might also possibly play some very soothing classical music that is played in the key that you desire. For instance, if you are working on problems of the thyroid, kidneys, spleen, or color in the second chakra (orange), you might find some gentle, healing music in the key of D. Then again, the intricacies of the full musical composition might prove distracting. You will need to use your own best judgment, based on your knowledge of your healing friend. If your friend can meditate and remain centered, healing music in the proper key might be helpful.

Heightened Consciousness State:

It's important that both the energy healer and healing subject remain in state of heightened consciousness. That means remaining centered. Both parties will need to tune out external and internal distractions and stay focused on the healing process. The healing subject in particular needs to tune out all external distractions and tune out all internal thoughts and chatter, focusing only on the healing process and the healer's voice as a guide. The healer will need to move around a little, but should keep movement and talk to a bare minimum of what is absolutely necessary to the healing session.

Thought Forms:

The energy healer needs to creatively visualize the color of energy that is required to restore a weakened chakra. In order to do this, the healer needs to be able to look deep inside to manifest that color, using the third eye. This is not seeing in the normal physical sense, but seeing as seers do with insight. Once healers can creatively visualize inside themselves, they can project that energy outward to the subject as a target thought form. Think of it sort of like a telegraph signal. It's a message laced with energy. The message is partly the energy itself, but contains more than just the healing energy. The thought form contains the intent to heal. So for a thought form to become thought power and have transformative power as a projection, it needs intent.

Intent and Will:

The aura healer will need to focus intent on the healing process in order to project energy to assist the healing subject. This means consciously intending to project and heal with energy. The healer should visualize the healing energy reaching its target area and being effective. A strong sense of intent, then, travels with the healer's thought form, as the healer projects energy. The healer can drive this intent to its target area with the power of will. Our will center is located in our lower abdomen region and can be called on by digging deep inside to draw upon it. This is a conscious exercise of will, the inherent power we have to drive our thought forms with intent and power. You exercise your will center when you want to accomplish something in a transformative way, meaning with energy that you move or change in a creative way.

Ending the Session:

You should wind down the session by bringing your ailing friend slowly out of the state of heightened consciousness where your friend has remained centered, grounded, and focused in a quiet, meditative mode. You do not want to just shake your friend out of this state quickly and walk away. Your friend, after all, has been out of body and in an altered state for some time. That state has been tranquil, restful, and relaxing. Jarring the person back to the aches, pains, noise, and commotion of the mundane physical world of normal consciousness can be unsettling for anyone. So tell your friend in a quiet, monotone voice that the session is now ending. Tell you friend to return now to his or her body, beginning to feel the toes tingle and the legs returning to life. The rest of the body stirs to life now; and you can help by talking your healing subject through it. Just tell your friend that the feeling is returning to the legs, then the torso, then the arms, chest, neck, and head.

Once you friend begins to move about a little, you might want to discuss how he feels or anything that you have observed in assessing energy levels and energy healing. Your friend might want to give you some feedback, too.

You might remind him that professional medical attention is always a good idea, if he has concerns. You can also schedule another session of energy healing in a few days. It is not advisable to bombard a healing subject with too much energy at any one time. You could schedule sessions a day apart, but no more frequent.

Finally, you might want to make notes about your observations and the color of energy that you projected, also noting the chakra area that seemed to require the most energy assistance. These notes could prove helpful to you next time you meet with this friend for another healing session, although the condition of the human energy field changes all of the time. Nonetheless, the last concerns and needs of your friend might be a good starting point in your assessment of needs next time you meet with your friend for a healing session.

Chapter 6

Healing Energy

Healing energy is all around us and inside us. This is true of all people and other living beings, including our pets and plants. Energy is a gift of nature and necessary to sustain all life. Energy in our bodies is absorbed, processed, and transformed. Massive amounts of energy of various properties and practical uses run through our bodies, making us transformers of energy and self-regenerative dynamos. Consider the intricate neurological system of our bodies and the electromagnetic qualities of our essential being that is apparent to everyone who has felt sparks fly from their hands when touching another person. It is the force that makes us run as an efficient mechanism that seldom breaks down.

When any of the particular energies in our bodies is depleted or clogged in our system, then we experience an energy drain. Remember, energy is associated with the proper functioning of our chakras that govern the operation of our bodies, with each chakra responsible for the health and well being of specific areas of the body. Each chakra is associated with a particular color of light energy and needs this particular light energy to operate and transform the body. The chakras absorb and process the energy for distribution throughout the body.

We become depleted of sufficient energy to properly operate a chakra and its area of the body whenever we become sick. Chakras lose their power as a force within the body. They cease to spin with the same speed and elliptical pattern. They cannot do their jobs when their source of light energy is depleted. Sickness comes to us in many ways, but is always debilitating. We can contact a virus, injure ourselves, or become ill in a number of unforeseen misfortunes that are beyond our control as efficient health systems. These situations drain the chakra of its required energy.

Also, the body can become clogged with energy that is properly generated by the chakras, but not allowed to flow properly throughout our system. This is a like a river that becomes log-jammed with too little water slipping through the clogged areas of the stream and a massive buildup of water that stagnates in the area of the log-jam. We are like a river. Water, oxygen, and energy run through our bodies all of the time—or at least should do so, if we are healthy. We become constricted in many ways. It can even happen when we are emotionally traumatized.

Healing energy is a divine gift that we all receive freely. Energy in the form of light rains down from the heavens all around us for us to naturally absorb, process, and transform for sustained energetic life. The energy comes to us in many subtle colors of light. People who are knowledgeable about photography might recall that what we commonly call white light really has many different properties, depending on the particular light itself. In color photography, blue light is known by studio lighting experts to have at least six known hues. Light has many levels of intensities or frequencies that might also measured as vibrational waves. Yes, light is vibrational and energetic. That's why it's so important to us and all living things as healing energy.

You might recall how health clinics or retreats have long advocated putting sick people outdoors in natural sunlight to recuperate. Just sitting outdoors under the blessed sun has long been considered good therapy. In years past, it was a very popular treatment to send sick people to rustic settings to rest and recover outside in the sunlight. Today hospitals make efforts to make recovery rooms better lighted and brighter, a wonderful improvement from early hospital rooms that would often pull the shades and darken the room.

This isn't true only of people, of course. Plants couldn't survive a day without quality light, as anybody who's ever tried vainly to raise plants in artificial lighting or a dark corner could attest. While we do not practice photosynthesis like our houseplants, we nonetheless need natural light for its energetic, healing qualities. Notice how a sunny day naturally perks you up energetically and makes you feel better? That's not just an emotional reaction. The natural light energizes us and revitalizes us on all levels of our being including our physical body, mental body, and all the subtle bodies that makes us whole as energy beings.

All of the healing energy that energizes us and sustains our lives comes from the sun. This is a gift of nature that rains down to us from the seven divine rays. One aspect of the seven rays is their life-energizing property that we naturally absorb in sunlight. Light bends as it enters the earth's atmosphere into a spectrum of seven colors. These colors are red, orange, yellow, green, blue, indigo, and violet. This prism of light gives unique vibrational properties to each of the seven colors in the spectrum. These seven colors are absorbed by living beings and generate the chakras that govern and sustain their energetic health systems. Red light energy is associated with the root chakra in our bodies; while orange light energy drives our spleen area chakra. Yellow light energy powers the chakra that governs our solar plexus region;

and green light energizes the chakra that governs our heart area and thymus region. Similarly, blue light energizes the chakra that governs our voice region. Indigo light energizes our third eye and areas of the brow; while violet light energizes our crown chakra and higher spiritual consciousness.

Think of the chakras as swirling vortexes of psychic energy. They spin in a clockwise direction in a semi-elliptical orbit with a specific color of energy associated with each chakra. If they are damaged, slowed, stopped, misdirected, or clogged, then they cease to function properly. It might help to think of them as flywheels that spin in a specific orbital pattern, speed, and direction. If the flywheel's motion is altered in any way, the mechanism it runs is debilitated.

So it is with us. We need our flywheels in perfect motion for our mechanisms to operate at peak efficiency without stopping or slowing down.

Because all seven colors of the light spectrum are enthusiastically absorbed on diverse levels of our being, it's realistic to speculate that the seven colors with their unique frequencies operate within us in different areas. In overlaying the Eastern system of chakras with the major endocrine glands and organs in the body, it's reasonable to assume that different properties of light energy react in our bodies in different ways. Hence, the seven chakras are each given a color value that relates to the seven colors of light energy. Since the chakras or every centers in us seem to energize and drive certain areas in our complex body mechanism, it's reasonable to assume that specific chakras resonate with certain colors or frequencies of energy that come into contact with them. Why else would chakras (or some aspect within us) automatically process or transform energy within us to energize us? There seems to be a natural affinity with certain chakras or areas of our bodies for certain energy frequencies. Obviously, then, each of our chakras or energy processing stations resonates naturally to specific frequencies of energy that come to us. In this sense, our chakras are like energy transfer stations or transformers that take the raw power they need and convert it into useful purposes for their particular tasks.

Scientists for years now have been able to measure the different frequencies of different colors of light energy, just as they have been able to measure the different frequencies of sound energy. Each is unique, with its own vibration. It's reasonable to assume that each chakra in our marvelous bodies responds to a different vibrational level.

Unfortunately, chakras within us become damaged, slowed, or decayed to a point where they are not functioning properly. If the body area that a chakra serves is clogged with energy not flowing freely, then the chakra can chock, in effect, and slow down its distribution of life-sustaining energy. Body energy blockages can retard or even stop a chakra from its otherwise perpetual motion as a swirling vortex of psychic energy. Similarly, a chakra's orbit can become a decaying orbit with reduced speed and output as a result of trauma, illness, or injury that stresses it beyond limits.

In the case of an energy blockage, it's reasonable to assume that the chakra that processes and relays this particular energy to the clogged area of the body is shut down or will soon respond to the blockage by sending out less energy to the area. That's the way the body generally works, if you think about it. Energy that isn't going anywhere suggests to its relay station that there is a restricting road jam and that it would be counter-productive to send more.

Trauma also could tax a chakra energy center. Trauma comes to us in many ways. A physical blow can traumatize us to the point the body begins to shut down and not process energy. That rejection could encourage the chakra to shut down, since energy is not flowing in a productive manner. Stress can also traumatize us and affect the chakras in a couple of ways. Typically, trauma will trigger a body shutdown where energy doesn't flow properly and the chakra or chakras respond by shutting down. This is a feedback loop. In some cases that involve stress, the chakras will work overtime in response to the body crisis and become depleted of energy. Trauma can be physical or psychological, but is always debilitating. It tenses us up and bunches us up. Typically, trauma victims will curl up or bend over with everything tied in knots.

The proper functioning of chakras can be damaged in subtle ways, too. Since the chakras operate in the entire energy field including the subtle bodies that surround us, they are vulnerable to damage and illness that we experience as a spirit and a soul. Such damage at the level of the subtle bodies is hard to detect anatomically or physiologically, except that the anomaly will eventually impact our total being on all levels, including our physical body.

The best that we can do as chakra healers is to assist an ailing friend by observing what kind of energy is needed at a particular time and supplementing this energy level. We seek to stimulate our friends' natural self-rejuvenating system by sending energy to them. But we must not think of ourselves as an energy relay in the same sense of a direct current transformer operates. If we think of ourselves as their cure and source of energy, then we fall into the karmic trap of an enabler, who spoon-feeds a dependent friend without the friend ever becoming self-reliant again. No, our role is simply to jump-start our friend's own energy centers by focusing on which chakra needs energy and then sending that chakra the color of healing energy that is associated with it. For instance, the root chakra (at the base of the spine) uses primarily red healing energy. Any problem in the body areas governed by this root chakra would be aided by a healthy flow of red healing light.

Sending Energy:

After we have reviewed our friend's symptoms, read our friend's aura and scanned our friend as best we can, then we face our friend to begin sending healing energy. You can do this best in a seated position in front of your sick friend. You should both remain in a meditative state of heightened consciousness and perceptive awareness. Your friend can remain quiet and still with eyes closed in this meditative state; but you as the aura healer should assume an active meditative state. Your higher consciousness should be racing a mile a minute in a rapid beta brain wave pattern of super consciousness. You should be perceptively aware and focused, about to project your will. You will need to become very centered with intent.

Make a final aura reading of your friend's head and shoulder area, this time allowing yourself to drift deeply into a meditative state of higher consciousness and heightened awareness. Clear your mind and tune out all internal and external distractions. Just look with your perceptive awareness without intellectualizing what you think you see and trying to force anything. What colors of light do you see around your friend? Perhaps you see only green light with a little yellow. You intuitively know in this state of heightened awareness that your friend might be new to meditation and is really just concentrating hard. That might explain the yellow, if your earlier scans have pretty much ruled out the likelihood of third chakra problems in the area of the solar plexus region of the body. And if you have already scanned the fourth chakra and ruled out the likelihood of ailments in the region of the heart and thymus, then you might sense that the green in the aura does not reflect thymus or heart area problems. It could simply be that your friend is projecting green as part of an overall healing process internally, with the heart fully engaged in the full body treatment. Then if your same case profile, aura reading, and body scan have all determined some kind of disorder in the area of the throat area, you might begin projecting blue healing energy to assist the throat chakra, for example. An absence of blue in the subject's aura would be a dead giveaway to this conclusion, of course. Reading auras and determining what color of healing energy is needed in a body is not always simple, but can be augmented by a body energy scan, case profile provided by the subject, and an intuitive aura reading. Do not be afraid that your reading is flawed, since all energy of any color that you send to your ailing friend can be helpful to some degree. Sending a color of healing energy that is not depleted cannot hurt your friend in any way. On the other hand, the skilled aura reader attempts to send the exact color of healing energy that is most needed to supplement and stimulate the natural self-rejuvenation system in a friend's ailing chakra system.

The quick reference chakra chart on the following page might prove helpful to you.

Creative Visualization:

Your next task as a chakra healer involves creative visualization. In your active meditative state of heightened consciousness, you should begin to visualize inside you what color of energy you want to project to your friend. You do not exactly create this energy, but actually draw upon the light energy from all around you and inside you as a living being who absorbs, processes, and transforms energy as a natural part of life.

You can project any color of energy that you select, if you follow a few simple steps. First, you begin to visualize what color you want to send, taking into account the analyzed needs of your ailing friend and your understanding that every color of energy has distinct properties and healing powers to affect certain chakras and areas of the body. You do this by conceptualizing what color you want. Remember, you begin

COLOR	CHAKRA	HEALTH AREAS	OTHER ATTRIBUTES
Red	1st (base of spine)	reproductive organs, urinary tract, rectal area, red blood cells.	Sex, vigor, strength, intensifying love interest.
Orange	2nd (abdominal area)	Thyroid, kidneys, spleen, colon.	Stimulation, attraction, happiness, kindness, good fortune.
Yellow	3rd (solar plexus area)	Digestive system, liver, stomach, lymph system.	Confidence, comfort, intense thought, persuasion.
Green	4th (heart region)	Heart, lungs, thymus.	Wellness, growth, fertility, energy, finance.
Blue	5th (throat area)	Larnyx, thyroid, jaws, tonsils, mouth, speech.	Protection, calming, serenity, understanding, truth, sincerity.
Indigo	6th (brow area)	Eyes, brow, headaches, hormonal imbalance, developmental disorders..	Depression, transformation, ambition.
Violet	7th (crown of head)	Headaches, depression, imbalance, mental deficiencies, nerves, cancer.	Melancholy, piety, power.

Chakra Chart

the healing process in assessment with perception. Then you conceptualize. You achieve your goal of manifesting and sending a particular color or frequency of energy by creatively transforming whatever energy you have inside you and all around you into the color you desire.

This strong sense of desire is a magical element, without which no matter or energy is ever transformed. You exercise your desire with a strong sense of intent and a force of will. Intent comes only with strong grounding and centering to a still, quiet place deep inside you. In this place, your higher consciousness and heightened awareness give you the needed realization to transform the elements at your disposal. In short, any color of energy that we can creatively visualize in this state of heightened consciousness can be summoned and projected. Transforming energy and moving energy is defined as true magic or *magick*, as mystics of old have called it. Do not confuse magic in this sense with the sleight of hand trickery and deception that stage magicians employ for entertainment. This is true magic—the transformation and movement of energy at will. And every one of us can do this, with proper intent and force of will.

You can practice this by sitting quietly in light with your eyes almost shut in a meditative state. Tune out all external and internal distractions and focus only on one single objective—absorbing, processing, and transforming light in your mind's eye. Allow the light to slip through your nearly closed eyes. You might think of your eye lashes as little gates that the light trickles past. First you see only white light. Let it fill you, so that you see it brightly. When it becomes bright and all-encompassing inside you, then consciously transform the white light that you see to yellow light. At first, the light is very soft yellow. In time in grows bolder and more distinctive, so that you are filled inside you with bold yellow light everywhere. When you reach this point, transform the yellow light inside you to orange light. Again, the color orange might appear faint at first, but gradually becomes bold, solid orange. At this stage, transform the orange light inside you to red light. When the red light in turn becomes bright and solid red, you might transform the light insight you to black. In time, the light becomes solid black. All that you see is black everywhere. Black, you see, is a precursor of all colors. Consider this black inside you as a blank blackboard on which you can write anything you want.

So you see now that you can transform energy by color intensity inside you, using the light all around you and inside you. At first, you may need to go slowly through this process to achieve the color that you want to project to your ailing friend. You really can't rush the process. And when you can actually see the colors that you intend to visualize inside of you, then you can truly believe that you have the innate ability to transform colors that you desire.

Once you manifest the color of energy that you intend to project to your ailing friend, then you can project this particular energy to your friend with the power of your will. This is not the same thing as will power or being willful. Rather, it is projecting your thought form as an energy signal from deep within you. Mystics for centuries have known exactly how to do this. They consider our will center to be located in the area of our lower abdomen. So the process of projecting our thought form with force involves digging deep down inside us and summoning our inherent force of will. It helps to visualize that area of the body and calling on it to give you force to project outward. In our case, you are transmitting a thought form that is energized with a particular color of energy.

As discussed earlier, you can also burn a candle of the color of energy that you want to send to your ailing friend and even play the musical note that corresponds to the same wave frequency as the color you intend to project. You can also bathe your friend in this light by projecting color lights or positioning your friend in a room painted in this color. Any or all of these things in combination help. The best single thing that you can do, however, is to project healing energy from yourself to your friend. That color of energy is more alive than anything else, since it's coming from you in a highly charged, projected, and intentional manner.

One thing that helps in the final analysis is your intention to heal, coupled with your visualization of the healing energy reaching its mark and working wonders. Your creative visualization, it must be noted, should not end with simply visualizing the right color of light energy to send to your ailing friend. You must complete the healing process by visualizing your friend receiving the energy in the right place and putting it to good use.

Difficulties Determining Colors:

Do not despair if you experience difficulty in determining what color of energy seems to be lacking and what color of healing energy you should project to your ailing friend. There really are no wrong colors, in a sense. That is, you cannot harm anyone by sending a surplus of blue healing energy, if blue is not the color of the healing energy that is really most needed. Your friend will simply absorb the excess energy and process it.

If you are absolutely uncertain, you might want to project green healing energy, since that is the color of wellness and the color that the body often radiates when natural self-rejuvenation is in progress. Moreover, green healing energy stimulates the heart, lungs, and thymus. Many energy healers prefer to work almost exclusively in green healing energy, in fact. You can't go wrong in projecting green healing energy.

Also, you might try projecting blue light for protection and a calming influence, if you are uncertain what color to send. Blue energy is soothing.

Another approach, if you are uncertain which color to send, is to send a rainbow of color by picturing each of the seven chakra colors in your mind in rotation. The drill to learn how to transform color in our mind's eye works well here, like a sort of internal kaleidoscope.

As you work with a healing subject over time, however, you will eventually come to recognize exactly what color or colors of energy are most needed by your subject. Be patient. You cannot always get to the cause of a hidden health problem that easily, but will require many aura readings and body energy scans to really see what's needed.

Chapter 7

Various Modes and Techniques of Energy Healing

Many forms of energy healing are available to the chakra healer; and all of them will work wonders. In a sense, it matters very little what form of healing or combination of healing modalities you employ. Healing energy can take many forms, as we have seen, from sound energy to light energy. Once you gain experience in aura reading and chakra healing, you will undoubtedly find a modality and routine that works best for you.

Some people have a natural affinity for certain ways of working with energy. Some people, for instance, are clairaudient with a natural, psychic gift for acute hearing. For them, it might be natural to work with sound energy. Similarly, some people are clairvoyant with a natural, psychic gift for seeing deeply in the way a seer looks beyond the obvious, physical evidence. For them, it might feel more natural to work with light energy. Other people have a psychic gift of sensitive touch, sometimes called Psychometry. In their case, they might find it natural to work off the body in doing energy scans and body energy work.

It is presumptuous, then, to assume that all chakra healers might read an ailing friend's aura and then project colored healing light as the only approach to sending healing energy and stimulating that friend to heal naturally. Consequently, some of the major forms of energy healing need to be considered as options that can be used as primary healing mode or in combination during chakra healing.

Thought Forms:

The main delivery vehicle described for projecting healing energy in its many colors of light involves thought transfer. That is, the chakra healer creatively visualizes the needed color of healing light in his or her mind's eye and then projects it as a thought form. The chakra healer visualizes what part of the body or which chakra needs this particular color of healing light; and the energy hones in on this directional beacon. In that sense, thought forms can always find their marks. It's very much like magnetic attraction. You hold the image of the person and vital area on that person who needs this healing energy and pick up on this person's energy signature. This is truly karmic attraction of two people who connect on an energy level. You are connecting on a spirit level. Once you have touched this person's spirit and sensed this person's energy, you can home in on him by simply visualizing him in your mind's eye. That's what perceptive awareness gives you in a state of heightened consciousness, where all good energy healers operate. You have keen awareness on a spirit level and can sense energy signatures.

When you put intent into your thought form and empower it with the full force of your will by drawing on your will center in the abdominal area of your body, then you have put power into your thought form. Intent and will put force behind your thought forms. Your thought forms become thought power when you empower them in this fashion. This force behind your thought forms helps project them to your target area with impact.

Your healing thoughts carry a signal or message. The signal calls upon the healing subject to accept new energy for processing and to react to the stimulus by processing and transforming more healing energy internally for self-regeneration. This is a lot like jump-starting a car whose battery is low. The battery accepts the charge; and then the car begins recharging itself once it is reactivated. Our chakras as energy centers within the body become run down in the same manner and need assistance to resume normal operation on their own.

Thought forms and thought power in aura healing have the added element of healing energy attached to the signal. Otherwise, the healer is simply sending thoughts without anything behind them. In the case of the chakra healer, however, thought forms are loaded with specific healing energy, which the healer has manifested. This healing energy is creatively visualized within the mind's eye through creative visualization. Once the healer visualizes the color of healing light that is needed by the ailing body, then the healer projects that healing light as energized thought form.

Distant Healing

Healing with thought forms can be done at a distance, since thoughts as energy can carry directly to any subject anywhere with the speed and accuracy of an arrow. Think of your thought form as a focused beam of energy. If you focus your attention on where you want this beam of energy to go, it will hit your mark with pinpoint precision. You do not need to calculate direction, length, or trajectory. Part of the focusing process is to creatively visualize your target. Once the image of your healing subject is clear in your mind's eye, your target is locked into position. This is the karma of attraction. It involves your magnetic attraction to those who are near and dear to you. You are electromagnetically charged; and so are your close friends. There is a magnetic bond that allows you to find them anywhere at anytime, if you properly focus your attention. You can "feel" your subject, as you creatively visualize this subject in your mind's eye. And then your healing energy, like an energy signal that is specially encoded, races instantly to the subject that you have sighted in this manner.

You can use distant healing, then, to send your healing thought forms to your loved ones who need help. It is not important that you know precisely where they are, only that you visualize them and focus your healing energy to send as a thought form. As we have seen, energy can be encapsulated in many ways. Our thought forms work particularly well when distance stands between our loved ones and our healing hands.

You can encapsulate your healing thought forms with colored energy to assist your friend's most challenged chakra, if you know the area of the body that is most stressed. Of course, it is hard to assess specific energy shortcomings at a distance, when you are unable to see your friend and scan your friend's energy field.

Some daring people might like to attempt astral travel to visit their ailing friends and actually assess these energy shortcomings in person. Astral travel involves putting oneself into a meditative state of heightened awareness, with the conscious intent to leave the body and go to a specific place. It requires patience and practice. The astral traveler should develop the skills of meditation, creative visualization, and focused intent before attempting astral healing. Then one must develop a strong sense of will to consciously leave the body through a point in the body that seems most comfortable (the forehead, chest, or abdomen, for instance).

In astral travel, one learns to see with new eyes of awareness in a spirit body, instead of the eyes of the physical body. Seeing in this fashion is not much different from the sort of scrying that the healer does face-to-face in reading the aura, but will take practice to master. Working out of body will naturally be more difficult at first, but has the advantage of working in a spirit body that can go anywhere and do almost anything, defying the physical laws that limit our physical bodies.

Easier than astral healing or even astral travel is simple thought form transfer that allows any caring person to heal at a distance. Many times, of course, an energy healer will already have a clear idea about what energy field shortcomings need attention. This knowledge comes from prior examination of the subject, seeing the subject in your mind's eye, and your karmic connection to your friend. Simply visualize your friend and then project your healing thought forms. Complete the process by visualizing your friend actually receiving your healing thought form and then beginning to recover as a result.

Light Energy:

Healing thought forms are generally used to transfer light energy, since we normally see energy as light in our mind's eye. It would be possible, of course, to visualize energy in another form and project it with our thought power.

It is probably easier for most aura healers to work with light energy for a couple of reasons. First, we tend to see visually within our mind's eye. We are familiar with seeing even in a visionary sense as seers. The way we customarily see in a physical sense is with light refracted off objects. In this sense, our physical eyes are like cameras that capture light bounced off objects. This is light photography. It's the way we normally see. So even when we close our eyes and visualize creatively in our mind's eye, we tend to manifest familiar images.

The other thing that makes light energy such a comfortable format for chakra healers is that the body naturally absorbs, processes, and transforms lights of various colors. Each color has unique properties and healing potential within us. We can see that clearly, once we learn to read auras. We can acknowledge that certain chakras as energy centers within the body absorb and process certain colors of light energy. Psychics who can actually see the chakras can recognize these soft, subtle colors of energy at work in these energy centers. So by sending energy as colored light, the aura healer projects to the ailing body exactly which colors of healing energy the body requires at exactly the light wave frequency that color has.

Color Therapy:

Considering the various colors of healing energy of the individual chakras, it's attractive also to consider color therapy. We have seen how aura healers can visualize and transfer various colors of healing energy in thought forms. We have also considered the colors of light that can be projected by the aura healer as light energy of varying wave frequency, each with particularly vibrational characteristics.

Now we should consider how color outside the aura healer can be employed in color therapy. Many therapists and clinics now use color in therapy in this fashion with good results. The color can be projected from a color wheel, slide projector, or almost any light source filtered through colored gels. Similarly, the ailing person can be placed in a room painted in the appropriate healing color. The best color to choose, of course, is always the color that corresponds to the chakra associated with the anomalies. That will be the color of energy that is depleted and badly needed.

Colored candles can also be employed in color therapy. If the healing subject needs green colored energy, then use green candles. If the sick person needs red healing energy, then use green candles. The candles project the color of the candles to a degree, although not with the directness and impact of thought forms. Nonetheless, candles have been used in color therapy for many years. Chakra healers who use more direct forms of energy transfer might want to employ candles or projected outside light simply to supplement their own personal transfer of energy.

Sound Energy:

Sound energy waves can be measured with precision in the same way that light energy waves can be measured. The vibrational frequency of sound waves distinguishes what we commonly call the A note from the B note in the diatonic musical scale. In fact, we can even equate musical notes with the colors that are associated with healthy chakras as energy centers in our bodies. The wave frequency or vibrations of middle C on the diatonic musical scale equates to the wave frequency of the red light (associated with the root chakra at the base of our spines). The wave frequency of B on the musical scale equates to the wave frequency of orange light (associated with the second chakra in the abdominal area). Similarly, E equates to yellow light, associated with the third chakra in the solar plexus; and F equates to green light, associated with the fourth chakra in the heart area. Also, G equates to blue light, associated with the fifth chakra in the throat area; and A equates to indigo light, associated with the sixth chakra in the forehead. Lastly, the B note equates to the vibrational pattern of violet light, associated with the crown chakra above the head.

This chart is no longer metaphysics and the secret domain of the psychic healer. Modern physicists have long ago made these connections. After all, energy is universal. It comes in many forms. It can be carried by sound as easily as by light. The frequency or vibrational wave intensity defines the properties of the energy carried by the sound or the light. One of these properties is certainly healing potential.

To understand how sound energy impacts the body, we must consider harmonic resonance. Everything has a natural resonance to it, vibrating at a certain rate that is specific to it. Buildings even have a certain resonance. Motors certainly hum with a definite resonance that we can easily hear. When a motor is out of tune or running badly, then we can detect the difference in its humming. That is the same with our bodies.

Supporting the natural vibrational pattern of a healthy, living thing creates growth through harmony. Disrupting the natural, healthy vibrational pattern of a living thing creates dissonance and disease through disharmony. Friction creates dissonance. Going against the smooth vibrational pattern disrupts the harmonic field.

The key to good healing in any thing is harmonic resonance. Think of keeping the humming motor revving at a natural and comfortable pace that allows it to perform at maximum efficiency, without stressing the vehicle it serves. When your car is missing on one bad cylinder or sputtering badly, the whole car eventually slows down and can even stop running entirely.

So the sound vibration that resonates harmonically with the heart chakra can be manifested simply by playing the F note; while the root chakra can receive harmonic resonance by playing middle C. Harmony binds, builds, and strengthens. If you doubt this, consider how skyscrapers are imploded by demolition crews simply by setting up resonant dissonance to decay the building's structural integrity simply using the wrong sound.

The aura healer can use sound energy in many ways, as long as care is taken to use the correct note to stimulate the correct chakra:

B Note	Crown Chakra
A Note	Brow Chakra
G Note	Throat Chakra
F Note	Heart Chakra
E Note	Solar Plexus
D Note	Sacral Chakra
Middle C	Root Chakra

How the aura healers might choose to project the healing sound of one of these notes is partly a matter of personal preference and partly what works best for your ailing friend. You might like to play a soothing classical selection of music played in the key of the particular note that you need to project to your healing friend. You might even think that the music that you have chosen is healing and relaxing to hear. On the other hand, your ailing friend might be unaccustomed to remaining in meditative states and find the music a bit distracting with all of its intricacies. Remember that your healing subject must remain centered and focus without becoming distracted. On the other hand, your ailing friend might find the music very helpful to the whole meditative process. You'll have to determine this with you own best judgment and possibly by trial and error.

It is also possible simply to play the musical note that you want to project to a particular chakra. There are a number of ways to do this. You could play the note on a set of bells, a piano, string instrument, or other musical instrument. Perhaps you have a little flute and could play the note over and over, pausing a few second between each note that you play for your friend. You could even record the note struck over and over on a piano or guitar and play the recording for your friend. Be sure that the sound is not jarring and has several seconds of spacing between each rendition. Another option would be to carry a little pitch pipe to play the note for your ailing friend. Do it softly and in a pattern with a little spacing between each sound.

The chakra healer also can manifest the sound internally and project it as a thought form. If you can transform light into any color you desire in your mind's eye with creative visualization and then project it as an empowered thought form, you can do the same thing with sound. Simply hear the note clearly inside your head. When you are certain that you are hearing this note inside you, then you are ready to send it in a thought form. Think of it as a loud signal that you are projecting to your ailing friend. Put the full power of your will and intent behind it to drive it to the chakra that needs it.

Many chakra healers might simply choose to use sound energy as a supplement to their primary healing efforts. It's perfectly fine to project healing light energy of a certain color associated with an ailing chakra and then play the musical note that corresponds to that color to also stimulate the natural self-rejuvenation of that chakra. The sound of the healing note will resonate with the chakra that needs it, strengthening the chakra through harmonic resonance.

Intonation:

Another way chakra healers can use sound to help heal is with their voice. Since the voice can be used in many amazing ways to help heal, it really deserves its own discussion apart from sound as an outside stimulus. That is because the voice contains your own personal energy that you transform from the energy naturally inside you and all around you. You can employ a variety of techniques for healing, including chant, intonation, or even magical voice.

Our voice holds great power in many ways. We can use our voice to soothe and calm a wounded person to help that person heal. We can also use our voice as a guide to put a person into an altered state of heightened consciousness. The soothing voice can accomplish both, when we speak softly and slowly in a sort of monotone voice. The flatness and patient tone of the voice is important here, because we don't want to startle or distract a person who needs to become calm and collected.

In this manner, a slightly more powerful voice that remains also calm, flat, and soothing can become a magical voice for healing. Our voice, after all, carries energy with it. This is especially true when we power it with intent, the full force of our will, and creative visualization. In short, our magical voice accompanies our thought forms. Our voice resonates harmonically with the ailing body at the point our creative visualization directs it. Our voice is even more than musical notes, however. It is our divine gift of the breath of life. Like all gifts of spirit, it should be shared in a loving, caring way.

The magical voice is something that you should practice, even though it's a natural extension of you. It requires a depth of tonal quality from deep inside you and power derived from your will center in the abdominal area of your body. Magical voice is different from conversation or a soothing voice. It is a powerful voice that you need to reach deep inside you to muster and deliver. To be effective, you must be perfectly focused in heightened awareness.

You can also use intonation to project vowel sounds in a healing manner. Vowel sounds can correspond to the pitch of the healing notes. Vowel sounds have long been studied and used by music therapists to tone the body. The trick is to hold the vowel sound and let it reverberate, as you intone it. The vowel sounds, then, should be long and projected from deep inside you. Think of how an opera singer will reach deeply for a note and hold it. Similarly, the tonal healer reaches deep inside the abdomen to power the intonation from the will center. Consequently, the tonal singer as healer draws deeply from his or her lower stomach area to empower the message as a healing signal.

It is possible to improve the vibrational quality of your intonation also by singing from your mouth, nose, and throat. This is sometimes called throat singing; and it very powerful. Let the breath of life exit your body in this tonal singing by the throat, mouth, and nose simultaneously, creating an intense reverberation effect.

You can also chant to heal with your voice. In chanting, a person repeats a certain sound or expression and then extends and projects it. For instance, you could chant a certain musical note that you have associated with the energy that is most needed by an ailing friend. Or you could chant something like the person's name, if the needed healing note or corresponding long vowel is present in that name. Chanting might be less physically demanding than throat singing or intonation for some people, but can be quite effective if focused with intent and the power of the will.

Healing with Hands:

You can also use your hands to heal in much the way you use your hands off the body to access energy anomalies. In scanning the body to detect energy problems, the healer hands operate in a receiving mode without projecting energy. The hands in body scanning are sensitive to receiving energy signals from the body. When the healer uses these same hands to heal, the hands project energy to the ailing body to stimulate the natural self-rejuvenation of the chakra energy centers.

Think of your hands as sensitive magnets. They can push or pull, send or receive. When you consciously use them to send energy into the body, you will notice that your hands become very warm and may even tingle. If you do not feel any warmth, tingling, or sensitivity in your hands during healing, then stand up slowly in place and rub your hands together in a circle pattern until you feel some power buildup in them. Your hands are also like a double helix, with power naturally spinning through them in a spiral pattern.

Consequently, you may want to move your hands along the body during healing in small, slow circular patterns to move the energy that naturally flows in this fashion from your hands. Be careful to keep your hands a few inches off the body to avoid tactile contact. You are working in the etheric level just off the physical body. This etheric level connects the physical body to the subtle energy bodies that surround the physical core. Here you can best touch the energy level of the physical body and the total being at a point that is sometimes called the health aura level.

If you choose to deliver energy to your ailing friend with healing hands, then follow the approach used for assessment during body scanning. Only this time, consciously project energy from your body, working your way from head to spine from the back and then from head to toes from the front. Focus your attention particularly on the chakra area that seems to most need energy assistance, putting your full healing intent and power of your will behind your efforts to project energy to that location. Do not stay in any one place more than a minute or so, however. A little energy goes a long way, even though it's hard to see this at first. You don't want to bombard a person with too much.

In time, you will begin to feel a feedback response from the areas where you project energy. Your hands will tell you that the area is responding favorably to the energy stimulation by projecting back similar energy. A healing body responds in this manner, as Kirlian photography has demonstrated with radiation discharge bursts from areas stimulated with electricity. It's a natural response from a regenerative, living being that has the ability to absorb, process, and transform energy. What you will normally feel in feedback from an area that is responding energetically is a warm pulsing sensation or intensified tingling in your hands.

Water and Stones:

You could also use water and healing stones in your energy work. Both are historically used in energy healing to encapsulate healing energy from one person to be imparted to another ailing person upon contact.

In the case of healing stones, the healer creatively visualizes just what kind of energy is required and where it needs to be administered in the ailing body and then projects that energy to put into the stone held tightly in hand. This requires both healing hands to project the energy into the stone held in the hand and also thought power. The healer, in effect, is charging the stone. Beyond the more obvious projection of energy from the healer's hand to the stone as repository of that energy, there is also a more magical aspect to this charging of the stone. The healer is consecrating the stone, charging it with a particular intent. Consequently, the healer should meditate a moment on the intent and then bless the stone before charging it. The healer should visualize the person who needs this particular energy and also visualize the person receiving this energy in the chakra energy center that is associated with this needed energy. The healer might visualize the color of healing light that is most required by this ailing chakra of the ailing friend.

Once the stone is charged in this manner, it can be given to the sick friend to hold. Ideally, the friend would hold the stone tightly in one hand and meditate to absorb the energy without distractions. Energy is a property of spirit. Consequently, it is best to be in your spirit body to send or receive energy most effectively, so that spirit can respond and begin the rejuvenation process begun by the outside stimulation. This is spirit touching spirit.

The stone could also be laid upon the person's body area that is associated with the problem chakra. The person could also carry the stone around during the day or even sleep with it. But the stone should not be handled by another person or allowed to leave the intended recipient's direct contact until the healing energy is extracted from the stone. After that happens, the stone can be soaked in pure water, smudged with smoke, or cleansed with sea salt. This is sort of like deprogramming for a charged stone. You could also give it back to the earth as a gift repaid to spirit by burying the helpful stone somewhere. Stones are the bones of the earth, which we borrow from time to time.

Many stones are associated with healing. Yellowish citrine, for example, works on the solar plexus chakra and helps the digestive system. Violet-colored amethyst treats the crown chakra. Red agate builds strength. Bloodstone, a greenish stone, is associated with the heart chakra. Bloodstone, in fact, has been used to halt bleeding and cure fevers. The quartz crystal is a good all-purpose stone to use to program for healing since it is clear and will amplify, transform, and focus your message. It makes a good recorder crystal to store your message.

You might give the healing stone to your ailing friend after your aura healing session, so that your friend can use the stone afterward, drawing energy from the stone long after your have parted. You can also send a healing stone to a distant friend, if you know what sort of energy to put into the stone, depending on your friend's condition.

You could use water as a delivery vehicle for your healing energy. The idea is to magnetize the water with your hands to put healing energy into the water for your ailing friend to drink later. You could fill a glass of water or a glass jar of water and then charge it energetically with your hands in the same way that you energetically charge a healing stone. Place your hands directly on the glass or jar and focus your intent to project healing energy into the water. Be certain what sort of healing energy you are projecting, based on you friend's chakra needs. You might project the color of healing light that is associated with that problem chakra and then visualize the healing energy reaching your friend in this area and benefiting from it. Creative visualization should see the entire desired effect played out to successful completion. Then use your healing hands and thought power to energize the water with your hands. Don't put your hands in the water, but only on the glass that encases the water. And don't use plastic. A glass beaker works best.

Your friend could drink that water later or even bathe in it. The healing energy will remain in the water for some time, as laboratory experiments have proven.

Combination of Techniques:

Chakra healing can combine all of these energy healing techniques or be simplified to just reading the aura and projecting colored healing light by thought form. It's really a matter of personal preference and what seems to work best for your healing subject. In time you will discover what works best for you and your friend in a particular situation. Every one of these energy delivery techniques works every time. Energy is energy in all of its many forms. The forms really just define the delivery vehicle and not the energy itself.

Our task as chakra healers is to determine what sort of energy is needed by an ailing friend as determined by the chakra and then deliver that sort of energy required by the ailing chakra. For some people, it easier to think in terms of colors; while other people might find it easier to think in terms of sound. Our energy systems are all of this and much more.

Whatever energy we project to aid an ailing friend, we must always remember that our role is not to totally heal the friend. Our role is simply to assist the friend to resume self-rejuvenation by stimulating our friend's chakra energy centers. Ultimately sick bodies of living beings heal on their own naturally. All that we can hope to do is supplement the ailing body's deficient supply of ready energy and stimulate the chakra energy centers to begin self-rejuvenation. The chakra energy centers naturally absorb, process, and transform energy for healthy living.

Chakra healers, like all well-intentioned body workers, must recognize their limited role in jump-starting the healing process in ailing friends. After all, there is no way our energy work in their behalf can insure that they will recover. Nor can our stimulating energy boost be long-lasting without self-healing on the part of the ailing person, who must begin to process and transform energy throughout the body from reenergized chakra centers.

When a living being's natural energy flow is depleted, blocked, or otherwise curtailed by a damaged or malfunctioning chakra, then outside assistance might be needed. But the need should be temporary, since the chakra energy centers in the ailing person will need to become self-regenerative in order to sustain health and life. As energy healers, we supplement the ailing body's own natural supply of energy at these critical times and stimulate the challenged chakras of the ailing body to begin performing at peek efficiency.

The ailing subjects that we assist should also recognize the limited role of energy healers and personally assume long-term responsibility for their own health. Consequently, it is important that healing subjects be properly oriented and maintain a state of heightened consciousness during the healing session to realize their own dynamic role as self-sustaining transformers of energy. Energy healers should make every effort, then, to make healing subjects consciously aware of their personal role in their rejuvenation and not allow them to become overly dependent on therapy in their goal to achieve and sustain healthy energy flow internally.

Chapter 8
The Magic Behind Energy Healing

There is something truly magical about energy healing. Transformation takes place before your very eyes, as two people exchange energy in ways that revitalize an ailing person. A person who was once sickly and very low in energy suddenly becomes reenergized and begins internal self-rejuvenation. Because all of this exchange of energy and the transformation with that energy is invisible to most people, it almost looks like a magic act or some kind of trick, like a sleight of hand in a carnival act.

Energy healing, in fact, is magical—but not in the common sense. This sort of magic is real, not a trick or entertaining deception. True magic is the movement of energy and transformation. Energy healing involves both.

Furthermore, energy healing involves the manifestation of energy, color magic, projection of energy, creative visualization, thought power, power of the will, divination, plus magical intent and focus. That's not all. Energy healing also includes spirit bodies, self-rejuvenation, the unseen world of chakras and auras, and our mystical subtle bodies. This is all part of a hidden world in a mystical approach to therapy that is gaining credence even in scientific circles today. What we employ to do this sort of energy healing on a spirit-to-spirit level is natural magic, as we tap the universal energy that flows all around us and inside every one of us from people to dogs and trees. Consequently, this approach to rejuvenation can work on anyone and can be done by anyone with the right approach and practice.

Divination:

Reading an aura and scanning a body's energy field involves divination or the ability to see as a seer can see with more than physical eyes. In this sense, the chakra healer's approach to seeing is a little bit like crystal gazing, candle gazing, water gazing, sky gazing, or even tarot reading.

In aura reading, the healer gazes with physical eyes shifted out of normal focus, perhaps a little to the left. The aura reader enters an active meditative state of heightened consciousness with external and internal distractions muted and the higher mind activated. The higher mind is attached to our higher self and to our subtle spirit bodies and consequently operates in a faster, more powerful mode than our normal, analytical mind (commonly called the lower mind or brain). The higher mind is capable of insight and reaching new heights, as it extends the consciousness beyond the limited sphere of the physical body with its petty concerns. The higher mind replaces the normal five physical senses that form our perception in normal consciousness with perceptive awareness on a higher plane.

In gazing to read an aura, the healer uses the physical eyes (which are half asleep like the rest of the physical body) only as a directional guide. The sleepy eyes discern light hovering over living beings as energy fields. Then awareness does the rest of the seeing. The aura reader *divines* the energy around the body and interprets it internally. This is done with the *third eye* of awareness. Mystics often visualize this internal third eye as somewhere in the brow area, associated with the pituitary gland. In reality, of course, it is not part of our physical body, so much as part of our spirit body.

As the aura reader meditates on the energy and visualizes it internally in this fashion, the reader begins to interpret the colors of the energy field. All bands of light energy, as we have seen, have unique properties of wave frequency, vibrational patterns, and colors that are associated with them. The aura reader as *seer* internally discerns and interprets the color associated with different light energy.

Similarly, the energy healer who scans a living body with hands to sense energy anomalies uses hands as a guide, in much the same way that aura readers use physical eyes as a directional guide. But the hands are not used in a tactile sense to touch the body for normal feeling. The hands are moved slowly along the body a few inches from actual tactile contact to sense energy vibrations throughout the body, using *Psychometry,* or the psychic perception of feeling without actually touching. This is done with awareness in a state of heightened consciousness and cannot be done effectively if not in this active meditative state. As with aura reading, the body scanner interprets the vibrational feelings internally and visualizes what these feelings are in terms of energy anomalies.

Thought Forms:

Magical thought forms are different from other thoughts that people have routinely running through their heads. Thought forms are focused energy signals that are projected to a specific target or receiver. Consequently, they are energetically charged and purposeful.

Thought forms are the result of *creative visualization.* In creative visualization, a person visualizes what he or she wants to create and then manifests it as a fully formed image to project. This should not be confused with random or analytical thoughts that race across a person's mind routinely throughout the day. With creative visualization, people magically give form and purpose to thoughts inside their mind's eye. When the thought is fully visualized and manifested with form and purpose, it is energized and projected as thought power. This projected thought form then reaches an intended target or recipient as a signal that is energized with specific purpose. The act of manifesting this thought form and projecting it with purpose as an energized signal is magical. Transforming a thought into an energized thought form is magical; and moving that energy by projecting it to another person is equally magically.

Magical Intent

To project a thought form energetically to achieve change involves magical intent. Anyone can do this. We give purpose to our thought forms as a part of creative visualization. Part of the visualization process is to give form to our thoughts. The other important part is to give purpose or intent to our thought forms, determining where they will be directed and what they will accomplish. This determination is driven by the power of our personal *will center*, often considered to be located somewhere in the area of our lower abdomen. Digging deep down inside us, then, we summon the power to drive our intent forward with force. So it might help to think of your will center as a force center deep down inside you. It helps, also, to concentrate on this area to activate it, when needed to drive your intent forward as a projected thought form. When you do this, your thought form becomes *thought power*. Magical intent is combined with focus and the power of the human will to achieve magical transformation that is creatively visualized as a thought form and then manifested by the movement of energy. All change from form to energy or energy to form universally comes with force and desire. In people, the driving agent comes from the will center. Changing our thought forms to thought power is transformation or magical by definition. Projecting our thought forms involves movement of energy, which is also magical by definition.

Chakra Energy Centers:

Our chakra energy centers transform energy and move it throughout us to affect change. By definition, therefore, our chakras are magical. They absorb and process energy outside them and then transform it to affect change. They process light energy and sound energy to energize our bodies to give us both health and mobility. If you deny the existence of these unseen energy centers, how would you then explain bodily movement? What enables us to move an arm or a leg? Surely, such bodily movement involves muscles as pulleys and bones as skeletal structure. But what energizes our bodily movement? Medical science might refer you to the neurological system in our bodies. That's simply a way of acknowledging electrical impulses throughout the body. Where do we obtain these electrical impulses? Unseen energy centers that process and transform energy throughout the body offer a logical answer. Certainly, we do have an amazing range of motion and movement for a collection of flesh and bones. Isn't it magical?

Subtle Bodies:

Our total being is magical when you think about it in detail. Our chakras energy centers transform energy and move it throughout us to affect change. Furthermore, our chakra energy centers operate on all levels of our being. As we have seen, our total being includes unseen subtle bodies that encase us as spirit bodies. So our energy centers affect our higher mental consciousness, emotional body, spirit, and divine essence or soul.

Our subtle bodies that surround our physical body are light bodies without solid form. In a real sense, they are energy bodies. As we walk through life with the radiant auras that surround us, we are luminous beings of light with a solid core that grounds us. Without this physical core to ground us to the solid earth, we would float as light, energy beings without form and substance. We would be spirits. In truth, we are both spirit and physical substance, straddling the line between energy and matter. How magical!

What's truly magical is the way energy flows freely and cooperatively between our subtle energy bodies and our physical body. Chakras are present on all levels of our being, affecting all levels of our being. Consequently, energy moves freely from one level of our being to another—from physical to non-physical levels. This defines our divine essence.

What happens on one level of our being affects our health and well-being on another level. Mental anguish can affect our physical health. Psychological stress can traumatize our bodies. Similarly, physical anomalies can eventually damage our unseen physical bodies, as seen in our surrounding aura of colored energy. This is transformation through the movement of energy and therefore magical by definition.

Spirit Bodies:

We are spirit, as much as physical. Our spirit affects our physicality, just as our physicality affects our spirit. This level of transformation and change through movement of energy is unique to living beings. It is part of our divine essence or divine spark. The same may be said of dogs, cats, horses, pigs, pigeons, and dandelions, of course. All have auras, subtle bodies, energy centers, and spirit that operates simultaneous and cooperatively with the physical aspect of their being.

Natural Magic:

What's present and dynamic in all of us, then, is natural magic. It's all around us in nature and inside us. It's universal, affecting all living beings. Nature moves energy all around us and transforms everything. Nature takes electromagnetic wave energy from the sun and transforms that into many wondrous forms for our use. Light, for instance, is electromagnetically charged. Nature diffracts or bends light in a prism effect as it enters the earth atmosphere and transforms this energized light into various spectrum colors, each with unique properties based on the wave frequency or vibration of each. So the magic that enables us to absorb, process, and transform energy within us is natural. Nature offers all of us almost unlimited potential to transform energy that is given to us freely.

Consequently, everyone has the power to self-rejuvenate or help others to heal, as in aura healing. The energy that we receive with transformational characteristics is universal and given to all of us equally. We have a tendency sometimes to think of natural healers who heal with energy in a transformative way as special or gifted. Well, we are all special and gifted, blessed by nature with many gifts of spirit. These gifts should be shared. Light flows everywhere, wanting to fill darkness. We should not restrict our share of this light, but direct it where it is most needed and everywhere it is needed. It belongs to everyone.

Self-Rejuvenation:

We cannot overlook the transformative ability that is innate in all people to heal themselves. Often, we look to the healer, therapist, or medical doctor as the primary agent of healing. Most of the time, people maintain their own health and rejuvenate themselves by processing and transforming energy that they have absorbed. Even when stimulated by outside healing agents, sick people ultimate regenerate by absorbing that stimulus and transforming it internally with intent and power of the will. The proof of this is that people ultimately die, when they lose their natural will to live and desire to continue. People are not unique in this regard. Other animals and other living beings have the same potential for self-rejuvenation by transforming energy within them with intent and power of the will. This ability to transform energy within us with intent and power is magical by definition, of course. We take it for granted, but should treat it as a sacred gift of spirit, a divine gift.

Connecting Spirit to Spirit:

In sharing energy to stimulate health, we are connecting spirit to spirit. That part of us that creatively visualizes thought forms and manifests energy is spirit, not body. That part of us that attaches intent and power of the will to our thought forms is also spirit, not body. Our ability to project our thought forms empowered with energy is our spirit, not body. In receiving and processing energy internally, our chakras as energy centers occupy no specific bodily location, but exist on all levels of our being physically and externally as spirit.

In empathic healing and energy transfer, then, we are connecting spirit to spirit and moving energy on a non-physical level. This is truly magical, beyond what you can see and touch physically. It is the unseen world of spirit.

Mystics often refer to the world of spirit as akasha. It is a realm of unlimited energy potential, including all of the raw powers of the natural elements. It is an unknown realm of force, the primal force behind everything. The spirit side of our total essence or being relates to the spirit of the universe. They are the same.

When we heal empathically with energy as chakra healers do, we form a sacred bond with the person or other living being that receives our focused attention. Our personal egos and personalities take a back seat to our spirits, as we relate on a higher consciousness level. We share a natural karmic attraction, an electromagnetic attraction that binds us in a working relationship. Our dynamos become one. Our transformers connect. We are not strangers or alien in any way. We are whole in our union.

Healing, therefore, is a sacred act of sharing. It is returning what is borrowed to the whole. Some things are too precious and sacred to put a price tag on them. Our health is one such thing, because it is divine and connected. All of life is sacred and precious. Sharing our energy and our health, then, becomes a way of repaying spirit for what we were freely given in light and love.

Ethics of Magic:

Because healing is karmic connection that involves electromagnetic attraction, we need to observe ethics and rules of karma. We need to ponder how karma in application is the way we connect as spirit, being drawn toward certain acts of duty. Our spiritual need to help each other by sharing our energy is certainly an aspect of karma. The magnetic manner in which our spirits react to each other energetically represents an obvious display of karma.

Consequently, we must observe the rules and ethics of karma in not determining life decisions for another person. It is altogether too easy for an empathic healer to become personally invested in the healing process and the life of people we attempt to help heal. Those decisions belong to the ailing person. The will to live or die can only be made by the host body. It is an exercise of that person's will, intent, and higher consciousness. As healers, we cannot make decisions that affect the divine spirit and life essence of another person, but only offer assistance when requested. They must desire it.

When we force healing upon a person or bombard a person with prolonged energy stimulation, we are usurping that person's right to self-determination. When we attempt to heal a person whose black aura and every attitude tells us that this person is fated to die, then we are pushing too hard. This is unethical and violates the basic law of karma that a person cannot control the greater destiny of another person. Each one of us must deal with our own karmic destiny and weave our own fate.

The chakra healer who acts ethically and within the rules of karma will explain the process carefully to orient the ailing friend and then request permission to continue. It is unethical to enter another person's auric energy field without permission, touching another person's spirit.

The ailing friend should be encouraged to offer feedback and even tell an energy healer to stop at any time. Anything that makes an ailing person feel uncomfortable or uneasy on any level—psychologically, mentally, emotionally, physically, or spiritually, should be curtailed or redirected, at the desire of the ailing subject. As chakra healers, we seek only to serve our friend's need to regenerate. It is a sacred trust.

Chapter 9
Stimulating Self-rejuvenation

For an energy healer, stimulating self-rejuvenation in an ailing friend is a lot like jump-starting somebody's dead car. If anyone has ever enlisted your roadside assistance when their car wouldn't start, you know the drill. You ask them to open up their hood for you. Then you open up your hood. You put your batteries as close as you can get them, facing each other. Then you attach jumper cables to send energy from your battery to the battery of the car that won't start.

That's usually the first thing that people do when they come upon a stranded fellow motorist—offer them a jump-start. There might be more wrong with the car, of course. Everybody seems to realize, however, that the stalled car won't start if the battery is weak. Sometimes the battery is not the big problem, of course. Maybe the car will not start or stay running for other, more complex reasons. In such a case, a hapless motorist probably keeps cranking on the battery to try to get the car to start, thereby wearing down a perfectly fine battery. So the first thing that needs to be done in many cases is boost the battery's power to get the car running again.

Even new cars can suffer from a weakened battery. So much is dependent on the battery that it's sometimes hard to conceive how really simple it is for the battery to maintain itself and, hence, maintain the operation of the entire car. Batteries, after all, are little energy boxes that we rarely see, hidden under the hood. We don't show people our batteries, when they admire our car. We don't check them every day. We pretty much take them for granted.

Our internally batteries are a lot like that. We store energy and disperse it from our energy chakra centers. Normally, our chakras are pretty much maintenance-free, as they restore any energy that they expend in much the same way the alternator of our car works. Once your battery starts your car, your alternator takes over and rejuvenates your battery. Once our chakras expend energy throughout the body, they absorb new energy to process and transform from outside the body.

Weakened, stressed, or damaged chakras are especially challenged to re-energize, however. They might have been stressed by bodily injury on any of a number of levels including emotional, mental, psychological, or spiritual. They might be overworked in successfully dealing with internal trauma of some sort and find it difficult to absorb and process new energy as fast as they are transforming and using it throughout the total body system. Or the orbital speed and direction of these swirling dynamos of psychic energy might be decayed. That's when the chakras need a jump-start, much like a car battery that has been stressed. At this time, the chakra healer asks the ailing person to open up for an energy boost and sit facing the healer in a receiving position. The battery cables that we extend in energy healing are life lines to re-energize the chakras in exactly the form of energy they need.

As chakra healers, however, we must remember that we are only stimulating self-rejuvenation in ailing friends when we send needed energy, and not attempting to fill them with all of the energy that they will need. This is an important distinction, if you remember the analogy of the car. We jump-start a car with just enough energy to get the car going. The car then begins to run on its own; and the battery is strengthened the longer the car runs on its own again. You can wear down your own battery trying to sustain a battery that cannot take a charge or jump-starting a car with more complex problems. It's really the same with people. Once our chakras are stimulated and re-energized with needed energy, they can ordinarily respond again in a healthy fashion. Healthy chakras that are not stressed can absorb and process enough energy to transform the bodies they serve as energy centers. Healthy bodies, therefore, are self-regenerative. So all that we seek to do as energy healers is to supplement the challenged chakra in our ailing friend with needed energy that it can process In doing that, we stimulate the challenged chakra to begin operating again in a healthy fashion. It's just like sparking the battery of a weakened car. It takes just a little jolt to get it going. Then you want to remove the battery cables immediately.

The energy healer stimulates an energy response in the ailing friend by sending energy to the friend's weakened chakras. We know that energy stimulation will result in energy response from the ailing body, based on Kirlian research. Kirlian photography, developed by Russian scientists Semyon and Valentine Kirlian, basically measures electromagnetic field changes of the human body or other living things directly onto film, after stimulating the subject by high-frequency, high-voltage electricity. In addition to research by the Kirlians in the 1930s, work by Thelma Moss and Kendal Johnson of UCLA pioneered experiments with a low-frequency Kirlian device to study the energy bursts coming from biomagnetic energy healers' hands.

Such Kirlian photography is very different from traditional image photography that measures the light that reflects off objects. Normal image photography captures these image reflections on negative film through a camera lens. The Kirlian direct-printing process measures the discharge response of objects that are sandwiched between two electrodes and given a jolt of electricity. Curiously, even non-life forms that have been handled recently by human contact, such as a coin, show a sort of stagnant, uniform energy halo around them, when subjected to the electrical stimulus in the Kirlian process. Primarily, however, the camera measures the changing response of living life forms that are subjected to electrical stimulus in the Kirlian photography technique.

Perhaps the most amazing thing about Kirlian photography is its measurement of psychological states on the film, such as the natural healer's energy state. The Kirlian camera also has documented acupuncture points, measured the health of plants as a function of aura intensity, and physically documented bioplasma as the unseen fourth state of matter.

One of the original Kirlian experiments, which has been replicated in the West, captures on film the energy burst of the subtle bodies that surround a leaf. The experiment, known as the phantom leaf experiment, captures the energy field of a missing leaf—a leaf that has been physically dismembered. While the physical body of the leaf was removed, the aura energy burst of the leaf remained, showing the outline of the absent physical body. This documented research therefore verifies the energy field that surrounds life forms and also the spirit bodies that envelope the physical body. It demonstrates how the chakras exist outside the physical body, as well as inside the physical body, processing energy on all levels of our total being including subtle, unseen bodies.

Other Kirlian photography experiments measure the energy control that energy healers can demonstrate in directing the flow of energy, as it leaves their hands. The fingers of healers are placed between the electrode plates and subjected to electrical stimulation. The healers, however, are told to attempt to control the flow of energy that leaves their fingers in the resulting discharge, as though directing their energy flow in healing. Many healers demonstrate remarkable ability to control the flow of energy that comes from their hands in such contact-print photographs.

Not surprisingly, fingertips of energy healers in UCLA Kirlian experiments show a decrease in the quality and quality of energy burst after draining healing sessions.

Moreover, the Kirlian photography process can measure the color of energy bursts, which correspond to the basic colors of the chakras in the body. Here is proof positive, captured on film.

American psychologist Lee R. Steiner even used Kirlian photographs of her patients to diagnose their mental illness and measure their progress in healing. She captured their energy bursts on film before treatment and after treatment and described her observations in her book *Psychic Self-Healing for Psychological Problems*, which she illustrated with her own Kirlian photographs of patients. She looked for anomalies in the energy bursts of ill patients, noting lack of uniformity and ragged quality to the energy bursts of the ill. Recovering patients, on the other hand, demonstrated an improvement in the overall fullness, symmetry, and extension of their energy bursts.

Kirlian photography also demonstrates gross changes in auras during heightened states or states of arousal. Subjects would respond with great changes in the energy bursts that emanate from their body when startled by the killing of a plant leaf. Curiously, plants respond with the same emotional energy changes to such stimuli, according to research in *The Secret Life of Plants*. The book describes how researcher Cleve Backster hooked plants to a polygraph machine and then recorded their emotional outbursts to threats made to other plants that were near and dear to them. Backster found that even unfertilized eggs would respond with emotional outbursts to similar threats made to eggs from the same carton, even when the eggs were separated by distance. Backster's new research in *The Secret Life of your Cells,* compiled by Robert Stone, shows that every cell in our bodies seems to respond emotionally with sensitivity and understanding of the total body's overall condition, even when removed from the host body and separated by great distance. All of these electronic laboratory experiments measure emotional energy or energetic response to emotional stimuli.

Chakra healers in attempting to stimulate ailing friends with energy boosts must be mindful of their own supply of precious energy. Most people get their raw energy in the form of sunlight, which offers the full spectrum of colored light. Chakra healers are no different in where they obtain energy, nor in the way their bodies absorb, process, and transform light energy. One concern for chakra healer is that they should work whenever possible in natural sunlight during healing sessions, so that they do not deplete their own source of energy. The sunlight will replenish energy that the chakra healer expends and transfers to the healing subject. In this regard, it might be helpful to think of the chakra healer as a conduit of energy from nature, rather than the source of the healing energy. The energy healer simply filters the energy from its raw form in nature, processed and transformed into the colors of healing energy that a body needs for self-rejuvenation.

The ailing friend could absorb and process the raw energy from the sunlight, as well. Once the chakras are stressed, however, it may prove difficult for the ailing friend to absorb and process energy as quickly as needed for recovery. The chakra healer can speed the process of self-rejuvenation by stimulating the chakras with the kind of processed energy that they need for healing. The chakra healer drives that energy directly to the chakras of the ailing friend with thought power and a personal force of will. The energy that is used to stimulate the ailing friend's stressed chakras nonetheless comes from nature, filtered through the aura healer in an energized location. Ideally, the healing session takes place bathed in sunlight, then.

Energy drains on energy healers come with a lack of recognition of the source of healing power. The healer draws that power from nature, typically from light energy. Many healers who drain themselves in sending energy to ailing friends mistakenly think that they are giving of themselves and draining their own energy reserves to assist their ailing friends. As a result, many healers expect to feel energy drains and respond accordingly. In reality, the energy expended by an energy healer can be replenished indefinitely by nature. Of course, the healer should conduct healing sessions in natural sunlight whenever possible. The healer also would be wise to keep healing sessions short, so that energy is being projected to the ailing friend no more than 15 minutes at one time. That way, the ailing friend is not overly bombarded with healing energy all at once in one session, and the aura healer has time to absorb and process new energy internally.

The sending of energy from a healer to an ailing friend will trigger sensations in both parties. That sensation will be markedly different in bodywork than in thought form healing.

In healing with hands just off the body, energy healers will be aware of a heat buildup in both hands, as the hands are used in tandem as a double helix. In this sense, the hands are somewhat like the electrode plates of the Kirlian camera that sandwich a subject to be stimulated energetically. The energy in this case runs from hand to hand, with the healing subject to be stimulated between the hands. Consequently, the energy healer seeks to keep the hands on either side of the body as much as possible, while otherwise conscious of the energy buildup between the hands and bouncing off the hands in proximity of the healing subject. (It is not always possible to "sandwich" an ailing friend's body between the two hands of the healer. In such case, consider your right hand to be your primary hand to send energy.)

The energy healer in bodywork senses this energy buildup in both hands just being engaged in energy transfer in heightened consciousness. During encounters with areas of the ailing friend's body where energy anomalies appear, the healer will sense increased heat, tingling of the hands, sudden cold spots, or even emptiness. Emptiness might suggest a troubled spot, perhaps devoid of adequate energy flow in that region. That could suggest disease, injury, or simply a lack of energy in that region. Moreover, the energy healer in bodywork might experience sensations of hollowness where energy is low. This sensation also strikes the energy healer when encountering a part of the body that is void, as with an artificial limb where no energy flows. Tingling usually indicates that the energy healer has encountered a part of the ailing person's body that is energizing to deal with an illness or stress area of the body. That also might be interpreted in many healers as an intense heat buildup sensed in the healer's hands.

When encountering such anomalies, the healer might ask the ailing friend about that area of the body and whether the friend feels any sensation there, too. The instant when a healer senses a sensitive, troubled spot is key. At this time, the healer should attempt to understand the significance. Once the problem is identified, the energy healer can respond with more intense healing effort in that troubled area, as needed, by projecting just the color of healing energy that is needed, using the hands as both a guide and delivery method.

The healing hands of all energy healers are sensitive, although many healers may experience the same energy spots in an ailing body a little different. The key for all healers is to recognize any anomaly in the subject's energy field and then determine the problem with regard to specific healing energy that could be directed at the problem area.

The ailing friend during bodywork experiences somewhat similar sensations to the energy stimulation from the healer's hands touching the energy field. The ailing person will likely experience heat of the healer's hands throughout most of the healing session and tingling or sudden coldness at certain times during the session. The ailing person should be encouraged to note any sensations during the healing session, using as few words as possible. This lack of verbal communication is meant to preserve the state of heightened consciousness of the healing subject, who remains centered, grounded, and focused on the healing process. In this sense, the healing subject is an active participant in energy healing.

Sensations are different for both healer and subject with thought transfer. In this mode, the healer faces the subject—both seated upright with feet squarely planted on the ground. The healer manifests the colors that are needed for healing energy and projects them at the subject in thought forms.

The sensations of heat, cold, tingling, and emptiness that both parties commonly feel in bodywork with healing hands are not generally present in thought transfer. These sensations are more associated with emotional energy, as the energy leaves the healer's body and is projected through the etheric level that binds the subtle energy bodies to the physical body. Consequently, the emotional energy buildup comes with using hands off the body in a non-tactile manner by touching the etheric level of the ailing friend, an area sometimes called the health aura. The etheric level is the connecting level between the emotional body and outer subtle bodies to the physical body.

In projecting healing energy through empowered thought forms, the sensations during the healing process are more subtle for both healer and subject. The experience should prove relaxing and calming for both parties. It should feel restful and tranquil.

Healers who project healing light with thought forms can sometimes experience a little mental fatigue at the end of the healing session, however, as the manifesting of energy in the required healing colors sometimes proves mentally taxing. Certainly the process of creative visualization and manifesting healing colors of energy involves the mental level of the healer. This should not be confused with energy drain, however, but only mental fatigue. In fact, the fatigue level should be minimal, if the healer is actively engaged in a state of higher consciousness and not attempting to manifest energy in a lower mental state.

Healers sometimes put undue pressures on themselves in attempts to heal by projecting energy and consequently believe that they must be stressed by the healing process. This is an illusion, however, since the healing process should be viewed as a sharing of energy that involves both parties and an unlimited amount of energy support from nature all around us.

In energy healing, two people touch spirit-to-spirit. This should be effortless and natural, as the energy we share is free for all. Nature's energy, with all of its amazing healing properties, is a true gift of spirit in the broadest sense. It is not all about us. It is not the sole domain of the healer. It is not something we can manufacture on our own. It is nature's universal gift to all to be shared.

In sharing this energy and touching spirit-to-spirit, we become connected and bonded on a karmic level. We support each other. We are responsible for each other. Our spirits have touched, as two magnets touch. The healer is affected by the touching almost as much as the healing subject. After all, we have shared our essential life force.

The energy healing experience, as experienced by both healer and subject, therefore makes us increasingly aware of the interconnectedness of all life. We are all spirits and part of a larger spirit that supports its many component parts. We are all connected by a karmic debt that each one of us has to repay. That gift is the sharing of energy and life that we were freely given as a gift of spirit. As our individual spirits touch in the healing process, we sense the way we are all interdependent and designed to help each other. Our essential life forms, our energy bodies, are interchangeable. We are all essentially the same, made from the same spirit energy.

Chapter 10

Treating the Subtle Illness, Based on Aura Reading

Treating illness with energy based on aura reading can be extremely subtle and slow. That is due to many factors, but primarily because illness can be subtle.

The chakra healer scans the body's energy field, looking for clues. Even after the healer has interviewed the ailing friend and reviewed a medical background profile offered by the friend, getting to the root of the problem can be difficult and slow. Medical doctors might refer to this process as diagnosis, of course. For the chakra healer, the idea is to get beyond symptoms as health indicators to determine the energy anomaly that could be affecting the healthy, normal flow of energy throughout the body from the chakras as energy centers.

Symptoms are like clues, but often inconclusive. Ailment in one area of the body can affect other areas of the body in many ways. Pain is not always localized, but can radiate to other areas of the body as associated pain. The body seeks to be a self-corrective mechanism and will even compensate for one weakened area. This can lead to other stress throughout the body.

When we begin to view the whole human body as more than a system of bones, connective tissue, and vital organs, we shift from a mechanical view of our essential being to a holistic view. What affects us emotionally on one level of our being can affect us physically, just as spiritual problems can affect our physical health. We are complex beings, with many subtle levels of existence.

The energy healer looks essentially at the energy flow in the body to determine whether anomalies in the body's "river" of naturally flowing energy indicate health problems. This can come with an accident, stress, disease, or a number of more subtle sources. We cannot reverse an accident or disease, of course. We can only proceed with the situation as it now exists in supplementing the body's weakened flow of energy and stimulating the body's own chakra centers to resume normal work as energy centers for self-regeneration. Many things traumatize or stress the chakras to a point where they are not operating correctly in producing enough needed energy. The goal of the aura healer, then, is really to determine which chakras need energy boost and to treat the health problem by projecting the type of healing energy that is naturally associated with the stressed chakra. Our ailing friend does all the rest.

Only the most advanced aura reader with special training in energy healing should attempt to treat anomalies of the subtle bodies that surround our physical body. These bodies, as we have seen, include energy fields that relate to our higher self and divine essence. The subtle bodies that are closest to the physical self—the emotional, mental, and causal bodies, impact our physical body the most in terms of physical health. Consequently, we will be dealing with energy anomalies in these subtle bodies as they become apparent on a physical level, treating the physical manifestation of the problem.

Energy colors that appear farthest from the body (a foot away or more) are generally associated with our outer spirit bodies and can be recognized as slightly different in color as the physical body manifestations of these energy colors. Remember that our chakra energy centers operate on all levels of our being, including all subtle bodies that surround us. The colors of energy that is most typically associated with the health aura and our physical well-being, however, are lighter and more pastel than outer colors of the subtle bodies. If we are healing on a physical or even psychological level with regard to emotional illness or mental fatigue, then we are looking close to the body for lighter, more pastel shades of colors that are associated with the physical body and the bodies that are nearest to the physical body and impact it in terms of health and well-being. Body scans for energy anomalies will only reflect energy flows on the physical level of the body, so can be performed to confirm aura readings of the physical health of an ailing friend or to replace aura reading, if the aura scans are proving difficult or inconclusive.

Projecting the specific color of healing light energy that is lacking, based on chakra association, is always the correct approach. That is always the ideal approach to supporting the chakras as energy centers within the ailing body. The chakras, once re-energized and rejuvenated, should be able to do the rest. As natural healers, we must trust the ailing body to heal itself, once properly rejuvenated. Our chakras, after all, are dynamic energy centers with specific area functions with regard to the whole body and its well-being.

When we are unable to positively identify which color or colors of energy are lacking in body, we still have certain options for treating illness in the body efficiently and responsibly.

Stressed Chakra Color Absent in Aura:

Ordinarily, we expect to find the energy color that is associated with the stressed chakra missing from the aura in aura reading. That is because the chakra that absorbs, processes, and transforms that energy for the part of the body that it governs becomes overburdened in times of bodily trauma and cannot supply enough of that needed color of light energy. In fact, by the time the chakra processes light energy that it has absorbed from outside the body, the energy is transformed by the chakra into something other than light energy. Nonetheless, bolstering a particular stressed chakra with colored light energy that is associated with it will re-energize that chakra with the processed energy that it needs to transform for use throughout parts of the body.

Severely challenged chakras often cannot generate sufficient energy to the parts of the body that are ailing. In truth, it is the chakra that is ailing, although the symptoms are seen throughout the parts of the body that the chakra serves as a regional energy center. Treating the symptom areas that the ailing chakra serves is a little like trying to fix a power plant generator problem by changing light bulbs in every house which the ailing generator serves. We must go to the source; and that is the chakra energy center. As we have seen, there are seven main chakra energy centers in our bodies; and each one powers a whole circuit throughout the body.

Chakras, as self-regenerative energy dynamos, often can meet the challenges of bodily trauma when they are stressed to the limits by absorbing more of the kind of energy that they need and processing more to meet the challenge put upon them. In times of energy blockages where the energy is simply not flowing properly, this approach will not work. The chakras in this case will slow down and may even lose their proper speed and orbit as swirling vortexes, somewhat similar to an engine's flywheel. When their orbits decay, chakras become damaged and ineffective. Chakras in such cases need to be re-energized to resume normal speed and shape of orbit.

The energy healer can adjust the orbit of the damaged chakra that has slowed down or stopped altogether in two ways. One approach would be to creatively visualize the damaged or immobilized chakra resuming its normally healthy clockwise orbit, swirling vigorously and rhythmically. The other approach would be to use healing hands in clockwise circles off the body in the area where that particular chakra is associated. Move the hands in sweeping, small circles clockwise with a rhythmic tempo, so that every circle made by your energizing hands is the same speed as the last circle.

In fact, it might be more effective simply to use your right hand cupped to make these small circles. Think of your hand as moving energy, because that is what it is doing. It is transferring energy and moving that energy in a small, clockwise orbit to restart the ailing chakra. If you elect to use your healing hands off the body to restart the troubled chakra, then visualize the color of energy that is associated with that particular chakra. Also visualize the chakra beginning to spin in normal clockwise fashion again.

If you sense difficulty in achieving your goal, consider that the chakra might have been totally stopped. In some case, chakras attempt to spin in clockwise orbits, but lacking speed will begin to rock backward in counter-clockwise orbit on occasion. You should be able to sense when the chakra is responded, because you will get a positive energy bounce back. This is particularly true when working off the body with healing hands.

Bodily trauma caused by injury, disease, or psychological stress might challenge the chakra that governs that area of the body, as well. A healthy chakra in a body that is not completely run down energetically can normally handle this level of stress and rise to this challenge by processing additional energy. Ordinarily, that is what happens in the body.

The healthy chakra that is able to meet the challenge of bodily trauma by processing additional energy will exude this color of energy as an apparent part of the aura. Most typically, healing people simply exude green, however. When you see soft green close to the body near the head and shoulders, you can assume that the body is healing. This would be especially true of the heart chakra, which is associated with green light energy. But if you see a little red close to the head and shoulders, you might assume that root chakra is producing extra energy to meet a challenge to its areas of the body. Often the overall healing process in the body is most visible in the aura as soft green, as the heart and lungs begin dealing with the bodily problem by processing more oxygen and pumping more blood to injured parts of the body.

When the aura indicates that the chakras are responding to bodily trauma and meeting the challenge by producing an excess of energy, then energy healing is often unneeded. This is the indication of a healthy chakra system, meeting the challenge energetically.

In such case, you have several choices, none of which is incorrect or inappropriate.

If you see the color of a healthy, working chakra that is meeting the challenge of the stressed area, then you might just want to project soothing blue light energy to calm the person who is suffering. This could minimize the level of psychological and even physical trauma that is associated with the illness. In addition, you could project indigo light energy to treat the nerves of the ailing friend. So your projected color could be a blue light energy with a tinge of indigo. Another approach would be to send blue light energy to calm the person overall, thinking of the holistic approach to treating the entire body system, followed by indigo light energy to treat the nerves, which might be stressed by the illness.

Sometimes, of course, the illness that is being addressed by the body's own energy system is not the only area of illness in the body. If the body is self-correcting in the sense that the chakra is obviously producing energy to deal with the challenge of one area of the body, the aura healer might observe whether there is another area of the body that is not coping as well. Pain, after all, radiates throughout the entire body. Associated pain might be present in another area, apart from the main problem area. Sometimes the body stresses itself in otherwise healthy areas to attempt to deal with problems that cannot be corrected elsewhere. We attempt to compensate to cope with pain that sometimes causes other parts of our body to become stressed by sudden overload and imbalance.

To determine whether there is more than one troubled area of the body and more than one chakra that needs to be addressed, the aura reader should review the information offered by the patient carefully, scan the body with hands off the body, and perform careful aura readings. Perhaps you will want to focus on the area of associated pain where the governing chakra is not meeting the challenge by producing enough energy. The longer illness or injury lingers in a body, the more likely that other areas of the body will be affected.

Sometimes the color of light energy that is most needed for the affected area of the body is present in the body, but still inadequate. You can generally read the aura colors as representing the energy that is most active in the body at that moment. And it is true that the auric presence of the right color to meet the challenged chakra is a good sign of self-regeneration on the part of your ailing friend. Nonetheless, severely pained or crippled people sometimes need even more energy that healthy, coping chakras can process.

If the aura healer opts to boost the energy level of a healthy chakra that is currently producing energy to meet a health challenge, then it should be done with the understanding that the projection of assisting energy should be slight. That is to say that the aura healer should not bombard the healthy chakra with an overload of complementary light energy, but only attempt to trickle a light extra energy to support the healthy chakras own output. Also, the projection of complementary energy should be brief—perhaps no more than a minute at most. Of course, treatments can be frequent, although brief each time. Perhaps brief treatments twice or three times a day might be enough, if spaced several hours apart. You want to avoid overloading the chakras with excessive energy, meaning more than the body system can handle at any one time.

Another approach for assisting a healthy, coping chakra would be to project colors of all seven major chakras, so that the ailing body is totally supported. Ailments can drain the energy of the entire body system, as the patient becomes weakened and stressed during illness centered anywhere in the body. In such case, the aura healer could manifest and project healing energy in each of the seven colors in succession—in any particular order. The ideal would be to project each colored light briefly, focusing the energy projection in the area of the chakra that is associated with a particular color of energy. Remember, too, that each chakra contains colors of energy other than the dominant color of energy that is ordinarily associated with it. Colors of energy that you project will have some affect on all of the chakras to a degree, although the basic color that each chakra needs to absorb and process for healing transformation will be the main color that is generally associated with that chakra.

No Particular Color in Aura:

There are many ways to interpret this condition. The first thing that should be considered, however, is that failure to see something doesn't mean that it is not present. Perhaps you are unable to see a color that is present and active in the aura. If you are new to aura reading and not developed as an aura reader, then perhaps you should carefully support your conclusions with additional scans off the body with healing hands and through interview of the patient to determine what seems to be wrong.

On the other hand, failure to determine what colors are present in the aura, with regard to a particular ailment, suggests that the chakra that should be charging up energetically to meet this challenge is unable to cope and needs help. That means that the aura reader should manifest and project the color of healing light energy that is generally associated with the chakra that governs the area of the ailment. This energy can be projected by thought form or by healing hands. Even with healing hands, however, the energy healer should attempt to visualize the color of light energy needed through creative visualization while focusing energy to the chakra area with healing hands. What makes chakra healing different from other forms of energy healing is that the healer manifests and projects the color of healing energy that is most needed by the stressed chakra.

If the ailment cannot be determined, even with body scanning and patient interview, then the aura healer who cannot discern a definite color in the aura could simply project each of the seven colors of energy associated with the major chakras. This can be done in rotation in any sequence, although it might be easier to begin with red focused on the root chakra and work your way up the body. Again, the aura healer should be cautious not to project any one color of light energy more than a minute or two.

Very dark auras:

On the other hand, a brown or black aura suggests serious illness or death that the aura healer should address. A brown aura generally describes a serious health condition; whereas a black aura describes imminent death.

Frankly, there is little that an aura healer can do about a black aura. Like a black cloud that hangs overhead, the dark aura is a specter that foreshadows what will automatically follow. Death is inevitable for all living beings. But death is only a transition from temporal life that needn't be dreaded. It is the doorway through which all people, plants, and animals must pass with as much dignity and consciousness as possible. For some people who have suffered long and hard, death is the ultimate cure. It ends their suffering and brings them peace, as it ends this chapter in their difficult existence. Chakra healers can help people with black auras by counseling them to meet major transition in their lives. It is not necessary to abruptly announce that the ailing friend is about to die. That is something the patient can resolve personally. The chakra healer can simply begin discussing transition as a normal part of living and the need in all people to face change readily as best they can. People who carry a black aura should be treated as evolving souls and addressed on a spirit to spirit level. Not all healing is physical. Not all transition is temporal.

Brown auras should be addressed by the chakra healers with urgency and diligence, as they suggest a serious condition that needs immediate assistance. People who are gravely ill, but still fighting for their physical lives, exhibit brown auras. The chakra healer who spots a brown aura should quickly determine the area of concern and the chakra or chakras that need energy assistance at soon as possible. The healer should discuss the patient profile in depth with the ailing friend, perform several intensive aura scans, and also conduct detailed body scans to determine where assistance is most needed. Time is wasting. There is grave urgency with a brown aura.

Chakra that won't respond to input:

Remember that chakras that are damaged, halted, rotating backward, or spinning out of normal orbital pattern need to be restarted properly in order to function on their own again. Consequently, a simple energy boost will not adequately set them into motion again. They have lost their self-regenerative capacity. Ordinarily, they can absorb and process complementary energy and cope with challenges that stress them during illness or disease. If chakras are damaged and not spinning correctly, however, they are no longer able to function on their own. They probably can't even process energy that you might project to them. Even if they can process the energy and transform it into healing energy to aid the body areas they govern, they will wind down as soon as they exhaust the energy boost. They have lost the ability to function on their own and will require repeated energy boosts from outside the body to assist them. In such cases, the aura healer will most likely need to use healing hands off the body to restart the damaged chakra.

The healer will need to sense whether the chakra is function properly or damaged. This can be done intuitively, with sensitive hands during a body scan, or by remote viewing out of body. It may be necessary for the healer to look inside the ailing person's body to examine the chakras in this case. The aura reader, already in a state of heightened consciousness, can send his or her consciousness into the body of the ailing friend. Yes, this is an out of body experience, as the consciousness of the healer travels into the body of the body of the other person to examine whether the chakras are spinning properly.

The chakras should be spinning clockwise in an elliptical orbit, making a slow revolution with regular precision. If one of the chakras is not spinning in this fashion, it is not generating healing energy. That's when the aura reader working off the body needs to cup his or her energized right hand over the area of the particular damaged chakra and restart it by making clockwise swirling motions just off the body. Don't touch the body, but stay inside the etheric plane just a couple inches off the physical body. And make very small, swirling motions with your hand (about one circle per second) with clocklike precision. Make these circles clockwise. Think of your moving hand as moving energy, because that's exactly what it is doing. It is like restarting the hands of a clock.

When you cannot discern colors:

Remember in treating illness as a chakra healer that you really don't see colored light energy with your eyes. You don't even really feel it with your hands. You sense it intuitively deep inside you, using something far better than eyes or hands. You are divining with awareness. Perceptive awareness is greater than sensory perception. It is keener, more alert, and more alive. It is an extension of your spirit, your divine essence. It is this part of you that connects you with every other spirit in creation. In this way, you are directly connected and in tune. Trust your awareness. Treat it with patience and reverence. It is our connection to all creation.

Chapter 11

Charting Progress with Follow-up Aura Reading

A conscientious chakra healer who wants to stimulate real health change should chart progress of an ailing friend and plan follow-up healing sessions, as appropriate. One healing session is not enough. If you do this sort of healing correctly, you will make your healing session brief and focused. Then you will repeat the session, building upon what you have learned and achieved in the last session.

Certainly you will want to maintain and update the case file on your ailing friend each visit. (See Chapter 5.) This updating gives you the opportunity to discuss your friend's medical history, noted symptoms, personal observations, and even family medical background. Remember that many conditions that are not considered "inherited conditions" have a way of recurring in various family members. In such "familial" cases, there is a noted tendency or susceptibility to a certain condition among family members. It could be a biological weakness. Consequently, you will want to know pertinent family medical backgrounds. This sort of information can be added in subsequent visits with your healing subject.

A good way to maintain an ongoing case profile is to keep your log of all treatments with the same healing subject in a three-ring binder. That way, you can keep pages in order and even insert new pages to record subsequent visits. You might want to keep the most recent visit with a particular healing subject first, with the previous visit recorded directly behind that recent visit. That way, you are always looking at the most recent information. The three-ring binder also allows you to shuffle pages into new order, as needed. You could easily keep records of several healing subjects in the same three-ring binder.

Don't hesitate to interview your healing subject again at the beginning of each new visit. This should be done prior to aura scans and actual energy healing. It's a good time to chat; and you can make the most of it by asking additional questions that have occurred to you since your last visit. Remember, your ailing friend probably knows more about his or her health condition that you do. This includes a lifetime of medical history. As you establish a rapport with your ailing friend, you should be able to carry on this little pre-treatment discussion without any awkwardness.

If all of these questions seems awkward to either one of you, however, you might want to prepare smaller questionnaires for each new visit. The questionnaires can be customized for each particular visit, as needed. Just determine what you want to know and then ask these questions (in writing if necessary). Always try to avoid appearing too personal, since this can upset many people and cause them to shy away from treatment. Simply keeping case files in a binder with a cover on it will give many patients a sense of comfort. It just looks more proper and more businesslike, as opposed to casual and personal.

Maintain a dated record of each and every visit with a healing subject and note any changes, observations, and impressions from each session.

Feedback:

During each treatment, you also should note any feedback that your ailing friend offers you. Do not write it into your notebook right away, but make a solid mental note of it. It could give you direction for how you want to proceed with the rest of the healing sessions. It could tell you what is working and what is not. It could help you identify troubled areas for concentrated treatment. So the feedback that you might receive from your healing subject could be pivotal in your approach to the treatment. After the healing session, make certain that you record this feedback in a report of that particular visit.

You also should end each healing session with a short discussion with your ailing friend. This is an opportunity to compare notes about how the session seemed to go. How did it feel? Does your ailing friend have anything to say about the session? The body is very sensitive to energy flow. It is sensitive to being touched with outside energy. It absorbs and processes this energy hungrily under normal conditions. Every cell of the body knows when something is happening anywhere in the body.

Our subtle bodies outside our physical body even feel this connection. We are all extremely sensitive to this touch. Sometimes it is difficult to articulate what the body feels, however. That is one reason why we want to try to connect to healing subjects on a spirit-to-spirit level, so that we can speak to that insightful part of a person's total being. Sometimes the physical self and even the analytical brain cannot articulate what is felt and what is happening throughout the total body system. Our higher consciousness, however, has a deeper awareness. That is one good reason why we want to put our healing subjects into a state of heightened consciousness during chakra healing. We need their awareness. We also need to be able to access that awareness for insightful feedback.

Keep Sessions Short:

There are good reasons to keep all of your sessions with one healing subject short in duration. Remember that the preferred definition of time for many modern physicists is *simply how long it takes for perceptible change to occur*. Once you perceive any change has occurred, you should consider the healing session complete. This can take just a few minutes. Your intake interview with your ailing friend, of course, will take a few minutes at the beginning of your visit. Then you will orient your friend and help your friend enter the proper state of centered, focused meditation for the healing session. Then you will take a few minutes to perform an aura reading, perhaps followed by a body energy scan or two. Then you will sit in front of your friend again and analyze your friend's aura once again, before manifesting colored light energy to project to begin the self-healing process of your friend. So the whole process, including the post-healing feedback session with your ailing friend might take up to an hour, but certainly should not take any longer under normal circumstances. The actual healing phase where you project colored light energy to assist your friend's challenged chakras, however, will require only a few minutes at most. Ordinarily, this phase—the key part of the chakra healing session, will take you less than five minutes, depending upon how readily you can manifest and project the light energy and direct it to the chakra that most needs it.

If energy healers bombard ailing subjects with energy projection longer than that, it could tire both the subject and healer. In addition, it could overload the weakened chakra with more energy that it can process at one time. Think of your energy projection as a burst of energy. It quickly reaches its target and is absorbed under normal circumstances. The ailing chakra responds by absorbing and processing the energy instantaneously and is strengthened to begin normal operation on its own under usual circumstances. When you jump-start a weakened car battery, you want to avoid sending energy to the car after it has restarted and resumed normal operation on its own. You want to quickly remove the jumper cables after the dead car fires up. It's the same with chakra healing. Simply send the energy that is needed to restart the weakened chakra and then disconnect the connection.

There are two ways that you can tell when the connection has been made and you are ready to stop projecting energy to your ailing friend. If you are projecting energy properly, you are projecting in thought forms that are empowered. You should be creatively visualizing in your thought forms what you want to send (manifested energy of a particular light color) and where you want to send it. The last phase of successful creative visualization is to picture where your thought form finds its target and how that target area responds to your thought form. So you should be able to creatively visualize when your projected energy is absorbed by the weakened chakra and how it responds. Remember, in a state of heightened consciousness, your heightened awareness becomes your all-seeing eyes.

You can also tell when the energy has been successful received by feedback from your healing subject. Words are not necessary. Your ailing friend can respond in many subtle ways that you will be able to perceive, because you are intimately connected on a spirit level. Often, the healing subject will appear satisfied or more comfortable. Your friend might make a happy, little sound. Sometimes the sound is internal, a harmonic resonance that your heightened awareness will perceive. This indicates that things are humming well again. Things are balanced and flowing properly. On an electromagnetic level, you can also feel a sort of energy backlash when an ailing chakra responds. It shoots out energy to the incoming source. You can feel this discharge, which is an automatic response. This is similar to the Kirlian camera subject that responds to an electrical stimulus with a radiation discharge that is seen on film as an energy burst from the subject after being stimulated electrically.

Assessing What You've Learned:

After you finish your visit with your ailing friend and part company, you should also record in your case file all of your observations and assessment. What have you learned from this session? This should help clarify the picture with regard to this healing subject, as you add your overall observations after each healing session. Here are some questions to ask yourself after conducting each healing session.

1. Are you seeing improvements?
2. Is the subject responding?
3. Are you able to read which color of light energy is lacking and what chakra needs help?
4. Are you aware of the condition of the chakra with regards to its orbital integrity?
5. It is spinning clockwise now?
6. Is it spinning in a constant pattern with approximately one revolution per second or so?
7. Is the orbit a healthy elliptical orbit?
8. Are the colors associated with this chakra returning to the chakra, as it begins to rejuvenate and become self-sustaining again?
9. Is your ailing friend appearing to be more energized overall?
10. Do you see any improvement in your friend's general health?

145

Refer to Medical Professionals:

If your ailing friend's condition appears serious, you should definitely recommend to your friend to consult a medical doctor or proper medical professional. Our friends deserve the very best health care that is available. This is especially true if your healing efforts do not result in any improvements. You should expect to see your friend more energized with chakra healing. If this is not happening—regardless of the perceived seriousness of the condition, you should recommend to your friend to consult a medical doctor.

Our goal in energy healing is to assist our ailing friend to begin self-rejuvenation. The specific approach of the chakra healer is to boost the energy of an ailing friend by supplement the specific energy of a challenged chakra and stimulate the chakra. This is clearly a supportive role. The chakra healer should not see his or her role as more than it is. We only assist the healing subject. All true healing is done internally by the healing subject.

The chakra healer's input, then, is complementary. It supports and assists. As such, it is a compatible supplement to any conventional medical treatment and should not be considered a stand-alone treatment in place of professional medical attention.

Repeat Treatments That Work:

The approach of the energy healer is intuitive. Consequently, the approach is to sense what works best through insight or divination. This is different from an analytical approach that is familiar to the scientific healer. As a result, intuitive natural healers will try different things to feel their way through the maze that is a health problem in a complex holistic system. A healer might try healing hands off the body, projecting different colors of light, or altering the intensity of the projected energy burst. A healer might try eliciting a lot of feedback;

and then try keeping a healing subject as quiet as possible for better focus. Some healers might try short healing sessions once a day; and then increase to sessions every twelve hours. As natural healers who operate with natural energy, aura healers feel their way intuitively and observe with awareness in a personal state of heightened consciousness.

At times, however, even an energy healer must stand back and analyze what seems to be working best to repeat what seems to work. This is only simple, common sense. You will want to repeat what works best. Sometimes that's only apparent by meditating on your past sessions, reviewing patient feedback, and comparing your patient reports from each and every session to date. Once you find something that works, don't waste your time doing other energy work. Focus only on the chakra or chakras that need energy boosts and stay with the delivery method that works best for you in projecting the right energy to supplement and stimulate the challenged chakras to become self-rejuvenating energy centers within the body.

Be Patient

We tend to think of our ailing friend who undergoes healing as a patient. The sick person must be patient for the treatment to take effect. The energy healer who seeks to assist an ailing friend needs to be patient, as well. Sometimes the improvement to treatment can seem instantaneous. Other times, recovery takes longer. Change sometimes occurs over many days or weeks and requires many treatments. This is a matter of inner transformation and cannot be hurried. Change takes place in its own good time. Perhaps it's better to think of the transformation time as duration. It might seem a long time for one person, but lightning fast for another. We all perceive time differently. We all perceive transformation differently. Forget about the clock. The only time that matters is the how long change takes to occur. All of your efforts as a chakra healer, if properly focused, will be helpful and be meaningful. At the very least, you will be able to calm your healing friend and give him reassurance. You might be able to reduce your friend's pain and anxiety. The very act of projecting energy into the body of another reduces stress. There are levels to stress reduction; and energy healers must learn to live with limitations.

Not everybody heals. Everybody most certainly has the inherent capability to recover energy levels under normal circumstances. But not all circumstances are normal. Sometimes chakras become so stressed and damaged that they find it difficult to resume normal operation as transformative energy centers, even with energy supplement and stimulation.

The wonderful thing about energy healing is that the patient healer can always try again. Our source of universal energy for healing is unlimited. Sometimes our patience is not, however. At these trying times, the energy healer might want to take a little time to meditate on the problem and the progress before trying again. Sometimes a temporary break in the action produces a breakthrough in results once treatment is resumed.

Taking ego out of the equation helps. The healer should not be discouraged for any reason of bruised ego, when results are not forthcoming. Natural healers must remember that they are only a conduit for healing energy. The important consideration is always the healing subject, our ailing friend who suffers and waits patiently for rejuvenation. As energy healers, we must remain patient, too.

Be Willing to Try Something Different

If nothing that you are doing as a healer seems to be working, you must be willing to try something slightly different. Trust your instincts. You approach this energy healing in a state of heightened awareness, so let awareness be your guide. You are connected to your ailing friend by spirit, so let spirit be your guide. Listen without ears and feel without touching. Sense what is happening and what might be needed.

If nothing seems to be working, you might just sit in front of your ailing friend with both of you focused in deep meditation. Clear your minds of all internal and external distractions. Cease internal dialogue. Shut down external stimulus and sensory perception. Focus your intent. Your mind should be blank like a clean slate in front of you. In this state of heightened consciousness, you are receptive. Soon something will appear on the slate in front of you. Trust spirit to lead you.

Maybe you have been trying to project one certain color of light energy, because that seemed to be the right thing to do. Sometimes our little brains get in the way; and we try to analyze things. Energy healing is a divinatory art form. It is a dance of spirit between two energy beings, trying to connect. It's not about brain work or rational analysis. It's about focused awareness in a state of heightened consciousness. This is the state of being where you can manifest, project, and transform energy.

Maybe you are not manifesting energy. Maybe you are not projecting it. Maybe your ailing friend cannot transform the light energy that you have been sending. Perhaps you should regroup and review your focused approach. If your approach is sound, perhaps you should try projecting a different color of energy. Be willing to start over and try something different, if previous efforts have been totally unsuccessful over a period of time. Remember, too, that problems that originate in one part of the body can affect other areas of the body. Maybe you have been focused in the wrong area or need to start the total treatment in another area first.

Am I Helping this Person Become Stronger?

The question to always ask yourself as an energy healer is whether you seem to be making your ailing friend become stronger. The healer, after all, works with natural energy and seeks to project that energy to strengthen an ailing friend. In some cases, the best that you will be able to do for your friend is to provide a feeling of calmness or ease the pain. Energy bodywork has been known also to reduce bleeding and treat people in shock. Energy that you project can have a soothing effect and help balance the energy flow in the body. Of course, the chakra healer also seeks to project a specific color of light energy to a specific chakra that is associated with that color of energy to strengthen and stimulate a challenged chakra under trauma when the area of the body is serves is ailing, injured, or blocked.

But there is a wise, noble tradition in healing that cautions against treatment when it might have an adverse effect. This dates back to Hippocrates, the father of healing arts, and is called the Hippocratic Oath. This is the oath that all medical doctors today swear. Actually, the ideal behind the oath is much older than scientific medicine, as physicians today practice it. The ideal dates all the way back to the roots of healing, when healing was considered an art form. Perhaps it's time for you to swear the oath and memorize it:

Hippocratic Oath:

"I SWEAR by Apollo the physician and Asclepsius and Gygenia and Panacea, invoking all the gods and goddesses to be my witness, that I will fulfill this Oath and this written covenant to the best of my powers and of my judgment. I will look upon him who shall have taught me this art of healing even as on mine own parents; I will share with him my substance, and supply his necessities if he be in need. I will regard his offspring even as my own brethren, and will teach them this Art, if they desire to learn it, even without fee or covenant.

"I WILL IMPART it by precept, by lecture and by all other manner of teaching, not only to my own sons but also to the sons of him who has taught me, and to disciples bound by covenant and oath according to the law of the physicians but to none other.

"THE REGIMEN I adopt shall be for the benefit of the patients to the best of my power and judgment, not for their injury or for any wrongful purpose. I will not give a deadly drug to any one, thought it be asked of me, nor will I lead the way in such counsel; and likewise I will not give a woman a pessary to procure abortion. But I will keep my life and my Art in purity and holiness. I will not use the knife, not even, verily, on sufferers from stone, but will give to such as are craftsmen therein.

"WHATEVER HOUSE I enter, I will enter for the benefit of the sick, refraining from all voluntary wrong doing and corruption, especially seduction of male or female, bond or free.

"WHATSOEVER THINGS I see or hear concerning the life of men, in my attendance on the sick or even apart from my attendance, which out not to be blabbed abroad, I will keep silence on them, counting such things to be as religious secrets.

"IF I FULFILL this oath and confound it not, be it mine to enjoy life and art alike, with god refute among all men for all time to come; but the contrary befall me if I transgress and violate my oath."

How Could Chakra Healing Hurt Anyone?

It's highly unlikely that anything done by a chakra healer who projects natural light energy to an ailing friend to assist that friend's self-rejuvenation could harm a person in any way. At the very least, you will boost his overall energy level a little and reduce his overall level of trauma. Occasionally, however, healing subjects might display discomfort with the energy healing session and become upset. This will probably be a psychological response, but must be treated respectfully. In such case, the healing session should be terminated. It is not the intent of chakra healing to cause a sick person to feel discomfort, if even emotional discomfort.

It would be permissible for the chakra healer to finish the aborted healing session in this case with a short discussion to elicit feedback from the ailing friend. It is fair to ask the ailing friend why the healing session caused discomfort and to review the process to attempt to address any unfounded fears or apprehension.

On the other hand, energy treatment that produces no results should be suspended and referred to other qualified healing professionals. It is the honorable role of natural healers to assist an ailing friend in healing any way that we can.

Chapter 12
The Role of the Wounded Healer

Generally speaking, only healers in good health should attempt to perform aura reading and energy healing. Just think how difficult it is to try to jump-start a car when you are drawing energy from a weak battery on the other end! What happens is that you just wear down the weakened vehicle by grinding down the starter and flooding the car. The two cars just grind away at each other, both getting weaker.

Weakened healers who attempt to rejuvenate others are about the same. Healers in a weakened condition should seek to strengthen themselves before attempting to lend strength to another. Healers with colds shouldn't attempt energy healing, nor should healers with headaches. They should deal with their own illness to regain their strength first.

And the reason for this goes even deeper. Weakened would-be healers must learn to cope with illness and overcome it personally before projecting themselves onto others. They have little energy to share and little credentials for sharing. They need to overcome their own challenges to gain inner strength of character as a true healer. The great strength of character comes from meeting the challenge and overcoming it. This is a heroic journey of self-discovery and overcoming personal obstacles. Overcoming obstacles gives a person inner strength of heroic proportions.

Role of the wounded healer

The healer who has overcome great personal wounds and rebounded with strength has insight and also empathy to share. Since energy healing requires insight and is essentially empathic healing, the wounded healer has much to offer.

The concept of the wounded healer is ancient and fills many of our most inspirational myths and legends. We see the wounded healer as a dynamic force in ancient Greek mythology, shamanic traditions, Arthurian legend, religious symbolism, and modern therapy.

Overall, what makes wounded healers effective is that they have suffered and continue to suffer after coming to grips with the source of their pain through much soul-searching. They have risen to the challenge and managed to energize themselves as functional people who are willing to share what they have learned and help others overcome similar challenges.

Chiron, the Wounded Healer

The oldest recorded legend of a wounded healer might be Chiron, the Centaur child of the father god Kronos (some say Zeus), who mated with the water nymph Philyra. The nymph tried to evade the great god by turning herself into a mare. Kronos then transformed himself into a stallion and mounted her. Philyra was disgusted to give birth to a creature who was half man and half horse, even though immortal. So she abandoned Chiron. This was innocent Chiron's first unfortunate wound from outside forces. But Chiron was raised by the sun god Apollo, the healing god. As a result, Chiron became a great healer himself and overcame his unfortunate psychological wound to help a great many people in his life

As an immortal, Chiron should have lived forever as a great mentor and healer. His misfortune continued to change his life, however. He was accidentally wounded by a poisoned arrow from Herakles (Hercules). The arrow was coated with the blood of the Hydra, known to cause wounds that could never heal. So Chiron would suffer forever, since he was destined to live forever as an immortal. He could never fully heal.

The god Zeus interceded at the request of Herakles and offered Chiron a chance for eternal peace with an end to his suffering. He could take the place of the chained god Prometheus, imprisoned and tortured for attempting to bring fire from Mount Olympus to mortals below. Upon his death, Chiron was honored by Zeus by placing him in the heavens with the constellation of Centaurus.

The story of Chiron, the wounded healer, has inspired people for thousands of years. Just recently, Chiron assumed an even bigger role. This asteroid or planetoid was discovered by astronomers in 1977 orbiting between Saturn and Uranus near the outermost edge of our solar system. Astrologers have given great significance to Chiron. They generally perceive Chiron as embodying the characteristics of both adjacent planets. Uranus is thought to produce awareness; whereas Saturn is thought to materialize awareness and bring it into material form. Saturn represents a sort of outer being. Chiron as a place in the heavens or in one's personal astrology chart, then, is thought to be a sort of shamanic bridge between space and time reality. This planetoid, which embodies the essence of the wounded healer, speaks for everyone who overcomes personal despair and suffering to reach out to others to help them endure the same sort of painful experience they have felt.

A Chiron wound, then, is an injury that will never totally heal, yet challenges the strong healer within us to learn and grow from coping with this sensitive area. After much personal struggle, Chiron wounded healers can help others by sharing their healing and what they have learned in overcoming their special pain

Classically speaking, the Chiron wound is an injury to one's instinctual nature and an injury to one's trust. This type of wound is caused by a stupid, thoughtless, careless act—most likely an accident of birth or youthful innocence. There is no one who can be blamed for intentionally wounding someone who suffers as the Centaur Chiron suffered.

The greatest pain or challenge one endures from childhood, then, eventually can become the source of great wisdom and healing powers for others, if you overcome these burdens heroically like Chiron.

Astrologers maintain that the position of Chiron in one's birth chart reflects the specific archetypical energies of the potential wounded healer within a person.

Amazingly, the discovery of Chiron in 1977 has ushered a groundswell of interest in New Age healing and holistic therapy. The emphasis has been on healing the whole person from the outside in, treating the psycho-spiritual aspects of our being as it impacts our physical health. The approach has been largely shamanic, which considers the spiritual wholeness of our being in terms of what ails us.

Types of Wounded Healer

We see many examples of wounded healers who help heal and strengthen others in our society today. Some of the best psychologists are often people who have overcome psychological problems as children. Some of the best dentists are people who understand pain. Some of the best allergists are doctors who suffered from debilitating allergies themselves as children. Some of our best physical therapists are people who have overcome physical shortcomings. People without speech often make the best teachers for sign language. Reformed alcoholics and drug addicts often make the best therapists or coaches in rehabilitation programs. These are people who have suffered and overcome great hardships. They continue to suffer, but have become strong enough in coping with their wounds to help others. They become excellent coaches, mentors, advisors, therapists, and healers. They understand and empathize. Moreover, they can share their insights on what it takes to deal with these special problems.

Shamanic Healers

The role of the shamanic wounded healer is ancient and appears in many cultures. In many nature-based folk religions, the shamanic healer is more than medicine man or witch doctor. The shamanic healer is the bridge between the people and the world of spirit and the bridge between their physical world and the unseen world beyond the physical. The shamanic healer in many such cultures is often a lame or injured person, most likely crippled since birth. The healer nonetheless walks between the two worlds and returns to his or her people with insight that will heal, teach, and strengthen.

Shamans were our first doctors, priests, and psychologists. They saw these functions fitting neatly together in the human body. To them, whole health included the body, mind, and spirit. They saw damage to the soul as dangerous to the mind and damage to the mind as deadly to the body. So they worked from the outside, entering the world of spirit on behalf of their people. Shamans would enter the dream world. They would commune with spirit. They would talk to the faces behind the forces of nature that impact our world. They saw a direct connection to our relationship to nature and our overall health and well-being.

Harmony between people and their natural environment was considered important by the shamanic healer. If nature was offended, the spirit world was upset. As a result, people would suffer from their alienation from the natural world of spirit. Obviously, they saw the living body as more than physical, but connected by layers of subtle spirit that could be visited as levels of reality approached through altered consciousness. To enter the spirit realm, the shamanic healer would begin with a vision and project himself to that level of being by altering consciousness. As with Chiron, the knowledge of the shaman's difficult journey produced healing insight.

Shamanism is probably older than written language, as practiced by indigenous peoples throughout the world. It has been passed down through the ages from generation to generation in rich, oral tradition. Many American Indian tribes have a rich tradition of shamanic medicine, often based in part on the concept of a wounded healer. The shaman ordinarily would not hunt, lead the tribe, or assume normal warrior duties. He was their healer, responsible for every aspect of their body, mind, and soul. Perhaps he was the one who was born with a defect or injured as a child. As he grew and overcame the challenge of this condition, his inner strength made him an ideal candidate for shaman to his people. His subsequent daring journeys into the spirit realm on behalf of his people opened him and made him vulnerable and therefore in a sense "wounded."

Even today, we have a rich tradition of shamanism in our modern society. If anything, shamanism is reborn in our time with healers who see the value of this approach. We see it in new psycho-spiritual therapy with an emphasis on the inner journey and connection to the spirit realm. The new interest in ecology and our environment speaks to this search for soul redemption and healing.

King Arthur's Grail Quest

The grail legend about King Arthur's deep suffering is familiar to many. At the center of this great adventure tale, however, is a story of desolation and emptiness. King Arthur's land suddenly falls into a strange, dark time. Spirits are low. Arthur himself falls ill. He dispatches his noble Knights of the Round Table in a quest for the lost Holy Grail. If Arthur receives the grail, his health will be restored.

The knights embark on perilous journeys, going in different directions. Where will they look? How will they recognize the Holy Grail, if they should encounter it? The knights encounter horrible, challenging ordeals along the way. They spend years in this quest, dying on the road. This is a difficult quest, to be sure. It is the quest to restore the soul and wholeness to the land and its people. Arthur feels the emptiness, but doesn't know exactly what is wrong. He knows that he lacks something.

Many people are like that. They feel a certain emptiness and alienation. They sense that they are empty inside, but do not recognize the extent of their desolation. Like Arthur, they mope and wait for someone to bring them what they need to restore their vitality. Unlike good King Arthur, they do not have champions.

Arthur's champions spent their lives searching for a cure to what ailed him. In the end, however, it was a shy knight named Perceval who unraveled the mystery and saved the land. The quest, after all, was really about knowledge and insight. Perceval had to solve a riddle. He found the grail castle, but then had to ask the right question in connect to a larger world. The question showed his humble vulnerability and willingness to admit to a lack of knowledge. In short, the knight on a quest to restore wholeness to the land had to display openness. This openness left the proud knight vulnerable, indeed, and left him open as though wounded. But this is the price of admission to this uncharted region behind the veil.

Perceval approached the grail castle the first time and failed, because he did not ask the question, due to personal shyness. He was unwilling to make himself vulnerable and open. So he left without the grail. When he resumed his mission and visited the grail castle again, he returned with humility and wisdom to admit he needed answers.

In this sense, Perceval is like the wounded shaman who opens himself to the unseen world of spirit and seeks to connect his people with this world of spirit and the knowledge it holds. This is selfless service to humanity. It is the quest for wholeness.

Perceval realized that the king suffered, as the land suffered. The two are connected. The king symbolized the people of the land, who also suffered. The quest is completed.

Legends and myths describe the inner journey of the soul. Many people thirst for the grail. They sense an inner emptiness and need to become whole again. They are alienated and alone. They suffer a spiritual void; and because of that, they suffer physically, devoid of energy. The grail is a quest many people can make to restore their kingliness and connectedness to the land and spirit. The search for wholeness can be a lonely, difficult quest for a sick person, however, without the aid of a good knight. The wounded healer can be that knight on a mission, unraveling the mystery of what unseen forces cripple us. The wounded healer seeks to restore our spirit and make us whole and healthy again.

Jesus as a Wounded Healer

For many people today, Jesus of Nazareth might be the ideal wounded healer, considering his suffering and sacrifice as a teacher and healer. Like shamans and Chiron, he was concerned with the soul and inner emptiness of his people, as well as their physical health and mental well-being. According to religious records, he was hunted as an infant by a king who feared his presence. As a result, Jesus had to suffer the knowledge that many innocent babies were slaughtered in his place in vain attempts to kill him in the cradle. Later as a young man he went on a journey of personal discovery and returned home to minister to his people. He taught and healed the sick in the open countryside along the sea, on hillsides, and in open fields. Always he taught with parables that were based on nature. And one of the great Jesus mysteries for Christians is that his suffering and death sentence gave followers a sense of redemption and new life.

Buddha as Wounded Healer

Similarly, Buddha went on a personal journey to find meaning and vitality in life. He was raised in a noble family and lived isolated in a palace. He left that behind as a young man and went on an odyssey through the countryside. Typical of the hero's journey, his odyssey ended in self-discovery. Everywhere he looked Buddha found people suffering and confused with an inner emptiness. So he ultimately completed his journey of discovery with an inner journey of self. He determined that people suffer because they are ignorant of their true nature and disconnected. One of his great lessons to his closest disciples took place under a tree. Buddha held a flower in front of them for them to admire. Slowly he plucked the petals from the flower and asked each one of them if they understood the significance of this.

What the Wounded Healer Can Do

Since the so-called age of scientific reason changed the way people typically see the world and their place in it, many souls have felt an inner emptiness and disconnectedness. This change in philosophical orientation has alienated humanity from nature and the spirit world. We have turned meadows into shopping centers and parks into parking lots. We have dumped our waste into the rivers and oceans. We have ravaged the forests and scalped patches out of mountain sides. This fragmentation and isolation has damaged our psyche, if not our soul. The proof is the sense of desolation and alienation that many modern people in our society suffer. These are open wounds that leave us feeling empty. How do we return to wholeness and feeling good again?

Knowing which questions to ask is a start, if we look to Perceval as an example. Also, approaching our problem with humility is a good start. Approaching the grail symbolically as a holy cure for our inner emptiness of spirit is another good approach. As the land suffers, so suffers the king and its people. We are so terribly disconnected and alienated from the forces of nature and its rejuvenating energy.

The wounded healer in modern society offers some hope. Such a person has suffered and continues to feel pain with understanding and empathy for others. It is not enough that a person has recovered from cancer, adjusted to amputation, or recovered from loss of a loved one. What makes wounded healers so amazing is that they understand how to make their lives whole again by restoring spirit, despite the open wound that will never fully heal. They have learned to meet the challenge of pain and cope with it, rejuvenating themselves with vitality and life. They have returned to wholeness, despite the gaping wound. And they have the understanding of how they did that, even if understood only intuitively.

We journey into spirit outside the physical reality with conscious awareness as our perception. Intuition becomes our feelers, as we grope about in darkness. What we bring back from the spirit realm is a gift of spirit that must be shared, as best we can. The wounded healer instinctively knows that and attempts to share this gift of spirit. It is an understanding of wholeness and connectedness, as much as empathy that makes the wounded healer useful to those who suffer. The wounded healer knows that there is more to us than our physical body. The wounded healer knows that non-physical wounds can make us totally sick.

So the wounded healer stands in front of an ailing friend without saying much. The empathic exchange between them is non-verbal and non-physical. They connect spirit-to-spirit on an energy level. Wounded healers, unlike all other healers, understand the pain and where it is found. They have been to this place and returned from the arduous journey, alive and wiser.

Energy healers who are true wounded healers can feel the emptiness and find the level of despair on whatever level of our subtle bodies it might appear. Because they are sensitive to this pain, they could be the ideal empathic healer. They will have an electromagnetic connection to their ailing friend, if they have experienced the same wound. They will have the same pattern in their energy field and the same hole in their subtle bodies somewhere most people cannot see.

The danger inherent in wounded healers, perhaps, is that they are not fully recovered and continue to suffer. Consequently, wounded healers must feel strong and whole enough to share their energy empathically in any form of energy healing and guard against personal relapse or personally spilling over into the energy field of the persons they seek to help. They must be strong survivors and whole enough to share their energy. As with all forms of energy healing, however, the healing sessions should be short enough to not stress either healer or the healing subject.

Chapter 13
Pets and Plants

Chakra healing works just as well for pets and plants as for people. In ways, it works even better. Pets and plants are naturally responsive to this sort of concentrated energy healing and will respond in kind by sending back energy to the healer. Consequently, the healing exchange is naturally symbiotic and mutually beneficial. Of course, this is also true of energy healing between two people, although pets often seem more attuned to natural energy exchange.

Chakra healing also works pretty much the same way with our four-legged loved ones, with minor differences. Similar to people, our pets have chakras that absorb, process, and transform energy that is specific for the operation of various areas of their bodies. Their chakras operate in multiple energy fields that include the physical body, but also extend from the physical body in subtle spirit bodies. Their subtle bodies that are located closest to the physical body most impact their physical body with regard to emotional and mental health. In fact, they have the same set of subtle bodies and the same set of chakras that absorb and process the same light energy as people utilize for chakras that govern the same areas physically.

Orientation:

One major difference in treating pets in an aura healing session involves orientation. You will not always be successful in verbally orienting your pet to the healing session, even though you might be able to convey some of the orientation non-verbally. Our dogs, cats, and horses speak without words, relying instead on thought forms. Of course, they tend to communicate with other animals in this fashion and might not be accustomed to communicating with people in this manner. Nonetheless, you might be successful in briefing them on the healing session ahead, if you combine thought forms with matching verbal confirmation and body language. Be sure to speak softly and slowly in a gentle monotone. Be focused in your thought forms by entering a heightened state of consciousness before orientation yourself.

Simply tell your pet that you are going to try to help restore health and vitality and that you will not touch them. You need to assure them that you are a helping friend who can guarantee their safety and security in your presence.

Don't worry about putting your pet into a meditative state of heightened consciousness. Unlike people, most animals are naturally grounded and centered and can enter a heightened state of consciousness quite easily. They just need to be relaxed and quiet to enter such a state. So make sure that they are calm, peaceful, and receptive of your presence. You might need to spend a little time sitting with them quietly or calming them with your voice. If they are agreeable, you might try petting them. Often it calms an excited animal to gently rest the palm of your right hand on their back about a third of the way down the spine from the neck.

Patient Profile:

Unless you are able to communicate telepathically with the pet about its health condition, you might need to gather health background information by talking with the owner and examining the animal. You also might be able to contact the animal's veterinarian, if you have permission of the owner and the owner clears this communication with the vet in advance. This is privileged communication, of course, but can be shared professionally once the veterinarian recognizes that you are doing some sort of worthwhile bodywork to assist the pet's overall health and the pet's owner agrees to release the information to you. If this direct approach does not work with the pet's veterinarian, perhaps the pet's owner can supply you with written medical records and a description of the pet's medical history and current condition.

Much has been written about the way animals apparently communicate telepathically with strong thought forms. Some speculate that people once had this ability, too, but lost it when our verbal languages developed and people become more vocal as a species. A few animal behaviorists, such as author Penelope Smith (*Animal Talk*) outline how patient people can learn to communicate telepathically with pets. Perhaps as an energy healer you can eventually communicate with pets in this way.

The difficult thing in attempting to help animals, of course, is that they cannot talk to you in a language you will easily understand. Consequently, you will need to carefully conduct your aura reading and body energy scans to augment the medical history and symptoms which seem apparent to you and the pet's owner.

Wiggling and Squirming:

Even though pets can easily ground, center, and focus themselves, you might find that nervous pets tends to fidget and move around a lot during a healing session. They might settle down, of course, after they become accustomed to you and what you are doing. Do not let this interfere with your healing session, but simply work around the situation by moving around with the pet. You will need to work with dogs and cats on the floor anyway. They will not perch on a chair for you, nor should you expect that. Let them be comfortable sitting or reclining on the floor. Sit on the floor next to them. Horses, on the other hand, will just stand in a place that suits them. Stand there with them. Adjust to your healing subjects.

Go Slowly:

You need to move slowly and deliberately, telegraphing your moves. This is true also of healing sessions with human subjects, but especially true of pets. Don't frighten or startle them. They will be wary enough. If you scare them, they will not be open to you and may even shut down to the point where their chakras will not readily absorb energy.

Do not stare into their eyes. That could be considered threatening. Show them that your hands are open and safe. Avoid sudden movements. Instead, slowly move from one place to another, so the pets know where you are moving ahead of time.

Begin with their Head:

It might be best to start with a body scan, since pets are so much more into their bodies than people. The best approach to beginning your body energy scan of a pet is to approach it from the back of the head. This is after you have greeted the pet face-to-face, of course and attempted to communicate with it verbally and non-verbally, showing it your empty hands and smiling face. Fill your heart with love and compassion. The pet will pick up on this. You might start with a gentle hug or soft head massage from the back (not facing the pet), if the pet seems comfortable enough with you to allow tactile contact. This sort of tactile contact is a good way to start with a pet, if you can.

Then put the palm of your right hand flat on the animal's spine about a third of the way down from the neck to the tail and rest your hand there for a few seconds to calm the animal. Project the energy of blue light to calm the animal at this point.

Then switch to off-body energy scanning with your hands a couple of inches from the animal's physical body. Begin with the crown chakra area above the head and slowly work down from the head with a hand on both sides of the body. Both of your hands should be facing inward to the body and facing palm to palm with the body between your hands. Focus your heightened awareness and remain centered and grounded, as you scan the energy of the body from head to tail, including all legs. Then work your way back up from the tail to the head again. You are trying to sense any energy anomalies in the body, which will seem to you like a warm spot, cold spot, emptiness, or tingling sensation. This is exactly the same as the way you scan the body of a human healing subject to determine energy anomalies that need to be addressed. Determine where the anomalies are located and what chakras govern these areas.

Some cats can be especially fidgety during body scans, but you will have to do the best you can. It might take several extra healing sessions before you can establish a body scan profile of a cat. Dogs generally sit still during energy scans. Horses are normally still during energy scans, too.

One thing for sure: You will be amazed just how responsive pets can be to energy work. They can sense the energy from your hands immediately. Generally, they will like this sensation and settle down considerably once they feel the energy from your hands. Their bodies seem to react immediately to this sort of energy work by sending back energy in response. That is especially helpful for assessments during energy scans.

Pets Make Good Patients:

Our pets are naturally close to spirit, because they live close to nature. Consequently, our pets are naturally grounded and centered and can focus quite easily. They live in the moment in connection with nature and don't clutter their minds with internal chatter. Consequently, pets make good patients for energy work. They can easily adjust to heightened awareness, because they live their lives in a state of awareness. They are accustomed to thought forms and body tuning. If you think about it, our pets seem to adjust and cope with sickness more easily than we do, bouncing back from health setbacks faster as a rule. Obviously, they are in touch with their body and the forces of nature. They seem to instinctively understand the self-rejuvenating potential of the energized body. We could learn a lot from our pets in this regard.

Symbiotic Relationship:

Our loving pets will return as much healing energy as they receive. They naturally send healing energy to those people and other animals they love. They do not have the same protective barriers that many people seem to erect. They are communal by nature and care for others. Dogs are pack animals. Cats live in extended families called colonies. Horses live naturally in large herds, caring for offspring regardless of parentage. When people enter their lives, it's typical for these animals to adopt us into their animal families and feel a part of our human family, as well. Our pets bond with us and share their love. That love is expressed in large part by their healing energy.

Pets can project their healing energy even easier than most people, because it's so easy for them to send thought forms. That's how they communicate normally. Their thought forms, like ours, can carry energy. If a pet is basically healthy, it will attempt to share its natural healing energy with loved ones.

And many pets that are loved by their owners display an amazing quality to love others. As a result, many dogs, horses, and cats are successfully used in health care programs to rejuvenate the energy level of people who come into loving contact with them. They are used in physical therapy programs, recovery programs, nursing home situations, group homes, and hospice. The one thing that is frequently said about the introduction of pets in these therapy situations is how energized and rejuvenated they make the people in these programs feel.

Minor Chakra Differences:

The location of chakras in most mammal pets is similar to that in people, with minor differences. In dogs, cats, and horses, the root chakra (red light energy) is located at the base of the tail. The sacral chakra (orange light energy) is located between the hips and over the spine. The solar plexus chakra (yellow light energy) is located in the center of the back at the base of the rib cage. The heart chakra (green light energy) is located in the center of the sternum in the concave center of the chest at the base of the neck. The throat chakra (blue light energy) is located between the scapulas at the seventh cervical vertebra. The brow chakra (indigo light energy) is located above the eyes on the forehead. The crown chakra (violet light energy) is located on the top of their heads between their ears.

The root chakra in these pets governs the spinal column, kidneys, stress responses, feet, and legs. It is associated with the adrenal gland, the psychological function of survival, and the will to live.

The sacral chakra in these pets governs the reproductive system and lower abdomen. It is associated with the gonads, desire, pleasure, and the will to feel emotionally.

The solar plexus chakra in dogs, cats, and horses governs the stomach, live, gall bladder, and upper abdomen. It is associated with the pancreas, laughter, anger, power of the will, and mental will.

The heart chakra in these pets governs the heart, circulatory system, arms, chest, and hands. It is associated with the thymus, loving, balance, and transformation.

The throat chakra of these pets governs the bronchial, vocal, lungs, ears, and respiratory system. It is associated with the parathyroid, thyroid, grieving, communication, expressiveness, and higher emotions.

The pets' brow chakra governs the lower mind, eyes, nose, and nervous system. It is associated with the pituitary gland, dreaming, intuition, imagination, visionary thinking, compassion, wisdom, and personality.

Our pets' crown chakra governs their higher minds. It is associated with the pineal gland, bliss, understanding, higher knowledge, holism, and the soul.

Plants, too

Plants also bond naturally with the people in their lives and willingly share their healing energy. They are even more grounded than our pets and totally focused on their connectedness to nature. When we consider how plants in dark rooms without sunlight will wind their way around corners in search of light energy, we gain a greater appreciation for the awareness of plant life.

Research by Cleve Backster and others in *The Secret Life of Plants* also verifies the empathic bond that plants have for people and other life forms that are near and dear to them. Their tests demonstrate that plants will respond emotionally to something happening to loved ones, even when separated by great distance. Now, that's empathy!

These plant researchers also have demonstrated convincingly that plants respond energetically to stimulus. You can demonstrate that to your own satisfaction with a little hands-on test of your own. Try cupping your hands on either side of a plant's leaf, so that your hands face inward without actually touching the plant. Keep your hands a couple of inches off the surface of the plant. Ground and center yourself in a state of heightened awareness. Focus your intent on sending energy through the palms of your facing hands, so that the energy passes through the plant. Keep doing this, until you feel your hands becoming warm or tingling. It should take only a few seconds to do this. The thing you want to observe here is the response of the plant. If you watch closely with heightened attention, you just might catch a plant responding enthusiastically. Perhaps you'll see it wiggle a little at the spot where it receives the energy. And people say that plants don't move! People are simply not watching with focused awareness.

Plants' response to stimulus is also demonstrated in Kirlian photography, which measures energetic bursts from life forms when subjected to electrical stimulation. In numerous Kirlian test cases, plants respond to energetic stimulus with energy bursts captured on film. The bursts are every bit as full and immediate as the energy bursts of people, who are similarly subjected to electrical stimulus in this fashion.

In some notable cases, the plants are even more responsive in their energetic feedback. The most famous of all Kirlian photographs is the "phantom leaf" experiment, in which the severed portion of a plant leaf demonstrates the same energy field as the rest of the physical plant. This also suggests that plants possess subtle energy bodies outside their physical body and are aware of them.

You will note in sending healing energy to plants that they send back at least as much energy as they receive from you. Try energy body work with a tree and see what massive amounts of energy the tree gives you in return.

In practical application, you might find this sort of healing-hands approach off the body better for plants, as opposed to projecting colored light energy in thought forms. Plants seem to like to have every leaf caressed energetically. Plants are sensual and very much into physical sensations, as opposed to thought. That is not to say that thought forms energized with healing light energy cannot be effective in helping plants heal. In fact, this might be the only practical way to reach some plants that are geographically distant to you.

Thought forms will work on plants, as with people or pets, because plants have chakra systems that absorb, process, and transform energy, too. They might not have the same seven major chakras as people and dogs, but they certainly have chakras that work for them. That is evident in the fact that plants naturally absorb and process light energy, even more naturally than people and pets. People and pooches might sometimes forget how important natural light energy is for good health, but plants are naturally aware of this universal law.

Orientation and Assessment:

Orientation and assessment in aura healing for plants will vary somewhat from the approach you will take with people or even pets. You should approach a plant in aura healing with reverence and quiet respect. Do not startle or shock them by bursting upon them and starting the healing process. Spend a quiet moment or two trying to making a spiritual connection with the plant. Make certain that you are grounded and centered in a state of higher consciousness. Focus your thoughts on the plant and quietly tell it that you love it and want to help it. Tell it that you are willingly sharing your healing energy.

Ordinarily you will need to assess the health condition of the plant through physical observation, followed by energy body scan. You might also know something about the health history of the plant. In many cases, the health problem of the plant might be obvious. You should be able to physically see whether the plant is drooping, drying up, weak, or has brown leaves.

Concentrate your healing energy on areas where the plant seems to be weak, shriveled, or brown. Apply healing energy to all areas of the plant that appear to need energy boosts.

As with people and pets, however, make certain that plants with serious health problems receive professional attention. Remember that plants need nourishing plant food, the right amount of water, the right amount of sunlight, and proper care. You owe it to your plant who lovingly shares its energy with you to seek outside professional care for it whenever its health is seriously compromised. Consult horticulturists, botanists, tree surgeons, greenhouse experts, and master gardeners.

Chapter 14

Practical considerations for energy healers

Since the bulk of this book has described almost unlimited potential for energy healers to influence change, it's important that we become grounded and practical in our application.

Be Sure You Are Properly Prepared

Be certain that you are properly prepared before attempting any sort of healing session. You will need to orient your healing subject and interview your subject to compile a patient profile of past medical history and current symptoms. You also need to prepare your ailing friend to enter a heightened state of consciousness by sitting erect in a chair with feet firmly plant on the ground, preferably with shoes removed. In short, your healing subject should be grounded, centered, and focused in a meditative state to receive the healing session. You should discuss your friend's condition, prepare your friend for the healing procedure, and encourage your friend to offer feedback if something feels odd in any way during the session (hot, cold, tingly, empty, or good). Tell your friend to remain quiet as much as possible to remain in the meditative state, offering comments only when feedback seems important with something really out of the ordinary. Then just a word or two will suffice.

You need to be certain that you prepare yourself for each and every healing session, too. You need to ground yourself, center yourself, and focus your awareness in a heightened state of consciousness. You need to be mentally alert throughout the process and ready to move around a little, if necessary, while avoiding excessive bodily movement and speech. Try to stay focused in heightened awareness. Your higher mind should be racing a mile a minute, if you prepare properly, and your hands should feel warm before you attempt any body energy scan or body energy transfer.

When you project energy in thought forms, you should be able to totally clear your mind of all internal and external distractions. You should start by seeing a clean slate inside your head. Perhaps that slate will look like a white slate, waiting for something to write upon it. Then through creative visualization and a conscious intent of will you need to change the white light inside your mind's eye to the colors of light energy that you need for the healing energy that is required by the challenged chakras of your ailing friend. If any of this doesn't come to you quickly or easily, you need to patiently focus yourself until it actually works for you. You can't hurry this sort of thing or fake it.

The same is true for aura reading. You can't hurry that or fake it, either. If you focus your awareness properly and scan patiently, you will be able to divine the colors of energy that are readily apparent in the aura of your ailing friend. It's pointless to hurry or guess

Work with an Assistant Initially

Maybe it would help you to work with an experienced aura reader at first, if you have difficulty reading auras. That person could confirm what you are seeing. Then you can gain confidence that the subtle colors that slowly come into focus during aura reading are actual aura colors manifested by the healing subject. Of course, you wouldn't want your "second" reader to lead you by telling you what you should be seeing. That would be directing you and not prove helpful to you in the long run. You might be talking yourself into seeing something that you really cannot see at this point, only because it was suggested to you by your guide. It would be better to verbalize what colors you see in the aura and then ask your second aura reader to confirm your observations. In that way, you can determine when you are really getting the feel for interpreting auras and a confidence to proceed with your readings.

Difficult Cases

You might especially want a second reader or energy healer to assist you with difficult cases. Combined effort of two healers who work cooperatively would be appropriate on cases that involve heart disease, cancer, aids, and other conditions that are progressive illnesses in advanced stages. That is not to say that you will be successful, even with the necessary involvement of medical doctors for primary treatment. Nonetheless, you can have an impact and should continue to creatively visualize the disease subsiding and normal health returning with the rejuvenation of chakras.

In addition to reading and scanning the aura for energy anomalies, the second healer can assist in projecting energy or off-body energy work by working at a complementary angle. In bodywork, the second healer can work from the opposite side of the healing subject, so that the two healers face each other with the healing subject sandwiched in between. The hands of the two body healers should work in tandem, so that the palms of both healers pretty much mirror each other with regard to location. In this manner, the two healers run energy through the body at the same location simultaneously.

For best effects with this approach, the right hand of one healer would be immediately opposite the left hand of the second healer. The left hand of the first healer would then oppose the right hand of the second healer. In that manner, the two healers begin sending energy back and force through the subject's body between them and can amplify the energy level. Picture the right hand as the positive magnet or the sending signal and the left hand as the negative magnet or the receiver. In a sense, then, the healing subject is perfectly sandwiched between two electromagnetic magnets that loop energy flow back and forth.

Similarly two energy healers can work together in projecting light energy to the challenged chakras of the healing subject by sitting next to each other and facing the subject as slightly different angles.

The cooperative healers can also read the subject's aura by sitting side by side and scanning the energy field at slightly different angles. In the case of body energy scans, the two healers should probably work separately one at a time to avoid reading each other while reading the subject's energy field. One healer can scan the subject off the body and then sit, while the other healer scans the body. Then they can prepare notes briefly before beginning either projecting light energy or body work.

Be Ready to Refer to Professionals

Whenever the energy healer finds anything that could be serious, the healer should be prepared to refer the ailing friend to professional medical doctors. Sometimes, of course, the healer will be asked to strengthen the overall health and well being of somebody who is not seriously ill. If in doubt, always recommend that the ailing friend consult medical doctors for professional examination and treatment in addition to energy work.

Don't Blast Friends with Energy Bursts

Just because you cannot necessarily see the energy that you project to your ailing friend and the impact of your energy boosts to your friend's own energy field and chakra centers, do not assume that little is happening. That could lead you to the mistake of blasting your friend with excessive energy. Often energy healers think that they should get immediate feedback and see results on the spot. When they don't recognize the impact of their invisible assistance, they respond with more powerful projections of energy over a lengthy period. Actual healing sessions (the part of treatment where you project energy to the healing subject) should be brief—no more than just a few minutes. Even twenty minutes can be too long.

The excessive energy can overload the challenged chakra, causing an energy imbalance. That is not highly likely, of course, but theoretically possible. More likely, healing projection that continues past five or ten minutes could exhaust both healer and healing subject. Remember, that the healing energy projection is a jolt or burst of energy that leaves the healer and impacts the healing subject. Any drain or jolt of energy can be a little disorienting and a shock to the body. The energy healer can always return to treat the ailing friend again later in the day or the next day. Short healing sessions spaced half a day apart or once a day are far better than one long blast of energy.

Work with All Life Forms

The aura healer should be willing to work with all life forms, including pets and plants. All life forms that absorb, process, and transform energy internally can benefit from chakra healing in the same way that people benefit from this focused form of energy healing.

In fact, energy work with other life forms will make you a better chakra healer. That is because you are exchanging energy on a subtle level with every healing subject. Our pets and plants give their energy to us generously and will respond rapidly to healing. They see it as a natural way to connect to others and connect to the spirit that binds us all. Consequently, they will readily absorb and process energy and respond in kind by returning energy. As a result, pets and plants make excellent subjects and will reward the energy healer with returned energy and speedy responses. This is true of all animals and plants. Anyone who has tried exchanging energy with trees, for instance, will recognize how sharing and generous they are.

Our pets and plants, therefore, offer excellent training subjects and generous patients that will prove rewarding to the energy healer in other personal ways. Any minor differences in the chakra system or subtle energy body field of pets and plants should not prove difficult for even the novice healer with a loving heart and healing intent.

Chapter 15

The Possible and the Impossible

Many amazing things are possible with aura reading and chakra healing, as we have seen. On the other hand, some things are not possible. For the natural healer who wants real results and a realistic approach to helping ailing friends attempt to heal, it's good at some point to sort the possible from the impossible.

As we have seen, the chakra healer is neither Superman nor Wonder Woman. Nor is the aura healer a magical magus. The healer is simply a catalyst for change. The real healing occurs within the healing subject. The energy healer simply relays energy to stimulate the self-regenerative process. The energy gift from the healer was never personal property, but a gift of spirit for everyone. The healer does not manifest the energy out of thin air, but collects available energy and filters it. Think of how a color filter works. That's what creative visualization can do for you as a chakra healer—provide you with a color filter to produce just the right color of energy that is needed from the universal energy that is all around you.

Normally, a body has enough energy to be self-rejuvenating with chakra energy centers that serve as personal transformers to monitor health in the body. Sometimes with illness, disease, injury, trauma, or energy blockages, however, the chakras become overburdened or even damaged to a degree to the point they no longer can maintain energy flow or even sustain their own precise orbital movement. Think of them as dynamos that spin around clockwise with a certain speed and orbital pattern to generate healing energy for the body from the natural energy that they absorb and process for internal transformation.

When these chakra energy centers are challenged to the point where they cannot operate efficiently with normal self-rejuvenation in the body, then they need assistance. That's where energy workers can help. Our approach in this book is to determine the specific chakra that needs help and determine the type of energy that chakra needs, based on the color of light energy associated with it. Anybody with a little training, patience, insight, and loving heart can help in this way.

Low Energy

Realistically, however, some things are easier than others when it comes to chakra healing. When the healer's own energy is low, it might prove difficult to project adequate energy to make any substantial difference on the part of the healing subject. While it's true that the healer draws energy from a universal source that is all around us, the healer nonetheless must be able to transform energy into the correct vibrational frequency or color that is required to stimulate and supplement the challenged chakra of the ailing friend. With regard to creative visualization and thought form transfer of this transformed energy, this becomes an internal exercise in manifesting healing energy of a particular type. Consequently, the chakra healer must transform energy into specific colored light energy. If the healer's own energy level is low, this might prove difficult. That includes instances when the healer is personally fatigued, ill, diseased, injured, blocked, or emotionally scattered. The healer could be traumatized mentally, psychologically, or physically in many ways that stress the healer's own chakra system and reduce the healer's ability to readily process and transform energy.

The severely weakened energy healer should not attempt to project energy. Any attempt could prove just too taxing on the healer and frustratingly futile for the healing subject. The holistic healer should heal himself or herself before attempting to heal anyone else. Then an honest attempt can be made on the part of the healer to heal another person. If that proves successful, then the healer can proceed more broadly.

In energy healing, we seek to heal one person at a time and focus on one person at a time. The healer who lacks the personal energy to project sufficient healing energy probably cannot gather focused intent to project the energy successfully. It takes a personal force of will to drive our focused intent in energy healing. After all, we must project the healing energy in a thought form that is directed at a specific chakra center.

Energy Blockages

Ordinarily, energy blockages within an ailing friend should not prove exceedingly difficult for the patient chakra healer to overcome with the right kind of projected energy. Of course, these blockages might require several healing sessions to unblock and get energy flowing normally. On the other hand, energy blockages in the aura healer might prove impossible to overcome. The healer must be able to transform existing energy that has been internally processed. Any energy healer who has internal energy blockages might have great difficulty amassing enough personally energy to project to an ailing friend. In such case, the healer should immediately realize that energy is blocked internally. The healer's hands will not readily heat up during body energy scans. Also, the healer will have trouble manifesting energy in creative visualization. In addition, the healer will probably feel drained or sense that a part of the body is not functioning well or with any sense of vitality. The blocked area may feel numb, dead, limp, or even disconnected.

Self-healing

In these instances, the healer might obtain the outside service of another energy healer to examine the personal chakra area that is blocked or begin doing self-healing meditation. One good self-healing meditation is to visualize healing energy of the color needed by the chakra that governs the blocked area. Visualize that colored light energy entering the chakra and surrounding area that is blocked, remobilizing the decaying orbit of the chakra if needed.

Another self-healing meditation involves creative visualization of a healing place or place of great personal power and safety where the healer can go to recuperate. This involves astral travel in which the healer focuses on leaving the physical body in an energy body. The healer visualizes a special place of personal power and healing and then projects both consciousness and energy body to that place. This is a place beyond time and space beyond the physical realm. Here the healer can focus colored light energy on the energy body. The energy body returns from this power spot and reunites with the whole body, bringing healing energy with it. This can be an extremely powerful out-of-body meditation for personal healing to restore energy to the entire body.

Trauma

Trauma is what often triggers energy imbalance in the body or chakra damage. Trauma can take many forms from physical damage to emotional stress. When the body is traumatized in any of a number of ways, the chakras as regional energy centers can be affected. Chakras can shut down, become backed up, or stressed to release more energy to the affected areas than they can normally absorb and process. Trauma, however, is not an impossible situation for the aura healer. Soothing blue light will relieve stress. The energy problems that trauma causes can be addressed over time by stimulating and supplementing the challenged chakras in the victim for self-rejuvenation to occur naturally.

Altered Chakras

Sometimes, however, traumatized chakras decay or become damaged in such a way they can no longer function properly, even with outside energy stimulation and supplemental energy. Even this situation is not impossible for the focused chakra healer who can reestablish the decayed orbit of the chakra. The sensitive healer must make energy contact with the chakra, most typically with the hands just off the body, and make an electromagnetic connection with the malfunctioning chakra. The healer will typically want to use the right hand and begin making small clockwise circles with this right hand just off the body where the chakra is believed to exist. In this way, the healer recalibrates the ailing chakra of an ailing friend by tuning the speed, direction, and orbital pattern of the friend's chakra to match the inner tempo of the healer.

It's a matter of becoming sensitive to one another and matching the rhythm of one ailing person to the energetic rhythm of another person. In a sense, the two match strides in a little dance of life to put the stride back into one tired dancer. Like everything else in sympathetic healing, this requires patience, connectedness, and focus. It might take several sessions and cannot be rushed or faked. Both parties, if properly connected in spirit during the energy exchange, will know the instant the ailing chakra is put back into proper working order.

The Badly Injured

Badly injured people or pets, however, need immediate professional medical attention. This is something that the energy healer should readily spot and facilitate by either transporting the injured friend to medical care or referring the friend to medical professionals. Natural healers cannot take the place of medical professionals in cases of medical emergencies and shouldn't delude themselves or anyone else into believing that they can. Our sick friends deserve the very best health care and emergency attention that we can hope to provide.

Energy healers, on the other hand, can supplement the natural recovery of ailing patients, once they have been treated properly by medical professionals. As sympathetic healers, they can help their loved ones maintain good health. They can do that by sharing their energy to stimulate chakras of their loved ones to function in an active, healthy manner as natural energy centers in the body. Nothing an energy healer does to stimulate and supplement the natural energy of their healing subjects is harmful or counterproductive to routine medical treatment in any way. Rather, the healer's assistance is complementary to all other medical treatment in supporting the self-rejuvenation of the healing subject empathically without touching.

Additional Treatment

Chakra healers, like other energy healers, sometimes seem to think that stimulating and supplementing the natural energy of an energy-depleted friend is all that is needed for their recovery. We must remember, however, that people who have been devoid of energy ultimately suffer other problems as a result of listlessness.

Consequently, they will require special attention beyond sympathetic healing.

Often the next step is to get such rejuvenated people quickly back on their feet and in the care of a physical therapist. That's because muscle atrophy becomes a problem with inactivity. People who have been low in energy have even been known to lose their sense of balance and ability to walk and talk easily. The muscles need to be retrained and strengthened. A physical trainer might be required for body strengthening. The chakra healer, like all concerned empathic healers, should quickly turn over candidates for physical therapy to trained professionals to reestablish their friends' range of motion and body strength after a period of listless inactivity.

The Dying

Healers must realize that dying is a part of living, a natural transition from the physical world to the world of spirit. All creatures die. Naturally, it is sad to all whenever anyone dies early at a young age through illness or accident. It is natural for healers to want to resist the premature death of a loved one in their care, but unrealistic to try to circumvent the inevitable.

Certain signs will tell the skilled chakra reader when life if simply weak or threatened by severe health problems to the point where death is imminent. The concern and treatment of the healer does not end with either sign, no matter how grim. The type of treatment will change, however, based on these signs in the aura.

People who are seriously ill with life-threatening illness will generally exhibit a brown or gray aura over their heads. The severity of the illness can be determined by how dark this brown or gray cloud appears and how fully formed this cloud looks in the auric energy field.

People who are facing an almost certain death with a lack of energy exhibited in their aura will generally display a black cloud hanging over their head and shoulders. As death draws nearer, this cloud increases in size. In such case, there is little or no other colors that are readily apparent in the aura.

A black cloud of death in an aura doesn't mean that treatment should be discontinued necessarily—only that other treatment might be more appropriate. The dying need pain relief, calming, and help with transition.

The energy healer, upon reading a totally black aura of impending death, can project soothing blue light to such ailing friends to reduce their stress, pain, and fear of transition from this physical environment. It is good to remember at these somber occasions that death can be the ultimate cure for physical ailments that are irreversible. Beyond the physical realm, there is no physical pain. So death ultimately allows us to discard a pained, decayed physical body. Our physical body ultimately fails us all, whereas our spirit body as pure energy is immortal. This divine spark of life can never be extinguished.

Energy healers who comfort the dying also can boost the overall life force of the dying by projecting green light or even white light. This will not necessarily reverse the dying process or extend life long, but might buy a little extra time for a dying friend to take care of matters and ease into transition.

The concerned energy healer also can work off the body with healing hands by projecting energy directly into the body through the hands. Since many hospice patients experience great physical pain, it is good to remember that you can project energy with your hands directly onto the body and all over the body without actually touching your patient. Keep your hands just a couple inches from actual physical contact, as you work your way throughout the body with your hands or concentrate your energy work in strategic areas of discomfort.

There is no need to project healing energy on these occasions to any particular chakra. Rather, you can radiate the soothing blue light energy everywhere throughout the dying body.

The energy healer also can help the dying by helping them *internalize* the soothing blue light. This approach involves personal effort on the part of the ailing friend to creatively visualize and manifest soothing blue light. As a healer and a friend, you can help your ailing friends to close their eyes in a grounded, centered state of heightened consciousness and visualize blue light inside their mind's eye. Once they can visualize the blue light inside themselves, they can direct the soothing blue light wherever it needs to go throughout their bodies. This will give your dying friends comfort, pain relief, and a peaceful transition that they can readily internalize anytime they want. They will consider it a blessing in their waning hours of pain.

People who exhibit the brown or sickly gray aura should receive intensive and immediate treatment with the goal of helping them heal. Until the aura turns completely black, there is always hope that the brown and gray clouds will give way to brighter, more energetic colors in the aura field. In such cases, determine the challenged chakra based on colors absent in the energy field and body scan to determine areas that are troubled. An interview with the sick friend should help determine which body area or areas are suffering. Once you determine the areas of the body that are suffering, then you can begin to stimulate and supplement the energy of the challenged chakras that govern these weak areas of the body.

Do not spend more than a few minutes in actual treatment, but be prepared to schedule many short healing sessions for friends who exhibit brown or gray auras. Remember that brown and gray in the aura demand immediate, intensive treatment with a sense of urgency. You might schedule healing sessions two to four times every day, if possible. You might even enlist the assistance of another energy healer to assist you.

As with all serious illness, you will want to refer sick friends who exhibit a brown, gray, or black aura to medical professions immediately. Around-the-clock medical care or even hospice might be advisable. You can't help everyone to heal, but you can help everyone deal appropriately with health issues.

Chapter 16

Reading Energy Levels All Around Us

Energy is all around us everywhere we look. We have been focusing in this book on the presence of light energy in the body as necessary for good health. The light energy that is absorbed and processed in the body, however, is universally present and available to all.

Universal energy also is carried in sound waves, just as readily as light waves. As we have seen, the middle C in the diatonic music scale is equivalent to the color red in the light scale. Both red light and middle C sound waves carry energy that can effectively impact the lower chakra or root chakra in our physical bodies, the chakra that governs our legs and other lower extremities.

Electromagnetic fields surround everyone and everything in our world, including the world itself, as energy rains down upon our world from the radiant sun above us. As a result, everyone and everything is energized through the forces of nature. This natural energy is absorbed, processed, and transformed in all living things, providing living creatures with the inherent power to transform themselves and the world around them. This is a marvelous blessing, this cooperative use of natural energy, and provides us with many opportunities to make changes in ourselves and the world around us.

But the ability to absorb, process, and transform energy is not limited to people and animals as living creatures. Trees, flowers, and even rocks have this amazing ability to transform energy. Science, industry, and the esoteric community alike realize the ability of the quartz crystal, for instance, to transform, amplify, and transfer light rays that pass through it. This use of stones is evident throughout modern society in many applications.

Piezo-electric quartz sparks

Quartz technology now powers our watches and many other electronic devices. The *piezo-electric* principle inherent in crystal-equipped striking igniters offers us a technological demonstration of how we manifest the divine spark of life.

Hug a tree back

While it might sound Pollyanna to some people, hugging a tree means more than simply a love of trees. Trees can transfer energy and share their inherent energy freely with people who approach them properly. Energy is naturally shared in a loving manner with others in a loving manner couched in respect and reverence. Make contact with the tree and attempt to become one with the tree in order to share its abundant, transformed energy.

Our bond with houseplants

Your houseplants and garden flowers can be equally generous in the energy they share with you. Show them love and care; and they will do the same. Make contact with them and bond with them. As demonstrated in the experiments of Cleve Backster and other plant researchers in such books as *The Secret Life of Plants*, the plants around us naturally want to bond with us and share emotional energy with us.

They care for us and appreciate the care that they receive from us on a sentient level that many people do not understand. It's simple, really. They love us and want to share their energy with us to strengthen us.

Strengthening each other

Together, we can strengthen each other. There is more to this than simply watering your plants or feeding your dog. We share energy with every other thing in our world, as we bond and become one with everyone and everything in the world around us. We reach out with our energy field and project energy that we share. Now, we can only do this, if we are healthy and have this sort of energy in abundance to share. These abundant energies are apparent in the various light colors of the aura. Anyone who can truly see will recognize this, as they scan the aura.

Our lights shine brightly

It's hard to hide who we truly are and what we're all about. Our emotional energy, mental energy, psychic energy, and physical energy glow brightly in colors all around us as beacons of our true being. We spill out all over, either consciously or unconsciously. Naturally, many concerned beings choose to share energy consciously after they have gone through the personal effort of transforming it.

Sharing the music of our soul

In this sprit of sharing and healing our planet, it's just as helpful to energize our loved ones with our music. If you raise a joyful sound, the energy of your sound energy waves will radiate with others, stimulating and strengthening their own natural energy centers. We have seen how musical notes act favorably upon specific chakras, as the wave frequency of notes correspond with the wave frequency of specific colors of light.

Ancient wisdom

None of this is very new, of course. It has been going on forever and will continue forever until the sun no longer shines. Even the discovery of electromagnetic energy as universally present and pervasive is ancient knowledge. Science has recognized these electromagnetic fields everywhere for many years, while mystics have experienced them even longer.

The Cathars, mystic Christians in France and southern Europe in the late middle ages, were among the first religious groups to recognize colors of light and sounds as transformative gifts of the divine. In fact, they viewed the Holy Spirit as light. The Cathars were respected within the Christian Church for many of their mystic beliefs, but eventually exterminated by the Church of Rome for other non-orthodox views, including their strong belief in reincarnation.

A modern religious organization, Eckenkar International, continues to view colors of light and sound as the true source of divine love and power. Eckists manifest the color blue and the chant *HU* to radiate harmonically with the divine essence of the universe.

The ancient belief in light as manifestation of the divine is found in some of our most revered religious texts, including *The Yoga Sutras of Paranjali, The Light of the Soul* by Alice Bailey, and the modern *Book of Light* by Jack H. Abendroth. The persistent belief in harmonic, resonant sound as divine is documented in *Harmonies of Heaven and Heaven and Earth: The Spiritual Dimensions of Music* by Joscelyn Godwin.

Spiritual evolution as light progression

The amazing past-life regressions of clients by Dr. Michael Newton in *Journey of Souls* shows how many hypnotized people remember lives between lives when they dwelt in light bodies in a spirit realm. Under deep hypnosis, they all remembered a system of spiritual evolution in this spirit realm. They remembered living physical lives on earth and then returning to a spirit realm for review and possible reassignment as a learning process. As souls evolved from lifetime to lifetime, their colors changed. One after another of Dr. Newton's clients, when asked specific questions about possible life between lifetimes in a spirit realm remembered being colored specks of light amid a soul group of other specks of light.

Indeed, we are energy that is temporarily encased in a decaying physical vehicle we call our body. In truth, we are much more than this physical encasement, which is temporal. We are energy that is depleted from time to time and rejuvenated from time to time with outside stimulation and supplemental energy from the world around us.

Willingness to share

Our ability to share and receive energy that rejuvenates us is perhaps limited by our willingness to share and connect with others. Regrettably, some people find it difficult to share and connect with others in this fashion. Some sad people are so disassociated from others in the world around them in extreme cases that they become immersed in a hollow world inside them. The extreme example of this disassociation, perhaps, is the catatonic state of complete withdrawal.

At the opposite extreme, we see happy and healthy people who approach life with both arms open and hands extended in loving friendship. That posture leaves one potentially vulnerable, but remains the only approach that allows a two-way exchange to the opportunities and wonders life offers. Many cultures watch such body language to determine if a stranger's hands are open, palm out. Clenched hands, after all, can conceal many hidden dangers. Clenched hands cannot grasp another in friendship to exchange positive body energy.

Open Systems, Closed Systems

The inability or unwillingness of many people to open themselves to this exchange of positive body energy eventually weakens them as a closed system with limited outside rejuvenation. That is something to carefully consider every time you are reluctant to extend a hand to a stranger, afraid to pet a stray dog, or disinterested in caring for a dying bush. In our unwillingness to share our energy with the entire world, we are limiting our exposure to shared energy and the rejuvenating effect of outside stimulation gained in each exchange.

Chakra healers through practice in reading energy fields and projecting energy to ailing friends will eventually understand this principle very clearly. People who receive energy healing might begin to understand this principle of energy exchange in time, as well. The illusion that limits many people is the mistaken belief that energy healilng is a one-way process.

With that mindset, sick people become dependent with a victim mentality and might never grow into strong, sharing individuals. This potential dependency is something that all healers should watch carefully. They should caution their sick friends to look at the entire process of energy exchange as a two-way process and an open system that allows them to grow stronger through energy exchange with everyone and everything around them.

The beginning of understanding for many energy patients is their realization of the "bounce-back" effect of impacting the healer with their own energy, as they receive energy from the healer during a session. The healer can validate this two-way exchange with the patient by noting the energy that is received from the patient by the healer.

Energy is something to share

We share, because we care. We should share unconditionally out of love that is open and giving. Trust that the world wants to share with you.

The energy that we share is a gift of spirit and universally available for all. It is not something to squander and claim only for ourselves. Closed systems decay without infusion from the outside. Open systems are rejuvenated.

Please choose to be open and rejuvenated, sharing your energy with everyone and everything around you. You will be blessed and made healthy in the exchange

Chapter 17

Exercises

Exercises are offered here as learning devices. The chakra healer might find these exercises helpful in the beginning as a summary demonstration of the points in this book. The exercises can be used for practice. In time, you can discard the exercises as primers and operate on your own.

Some of these exercises can help a person experience and recognize the healing impact of natural energy from the world around us. Of course, a person must have an open heart, open mind, and open arms. In addition, such people must enter a state of heightened consciousness by shutting down the physical distractions outside them and inside them to enter heightened awareness. With practice, people can learn to enter this heightened state while standing or walking, as easily as when they are sitting carefully in a meditation pose. After all, we need to enter the world around us in a state of heightened consciousness and not simply enter this state in a vacuum alone in a quiet room. The quiet meditation room and meditation posture should be viewed as only stages in our learning process, traditional crutches that we should learn to live without as we advance. .

EXERCISE: *"Feeling Energy Waves All Around Us"*

NEEDED:
1. Loose fitting clothing, ideally with shoes removed.
2. Outdoor setting.
3. Quiet isolation is best.

DIRECTIONS:

This is a little like surfers who catch the wave or children who stand outside to catch the snowflakes in their ready, open mouths.

Simply stand outdoors, facing the sun in a state of heightened consciousness. Tune out all distractions. Become conscious of the energy rays that are raining down upon the earth and rejuvenating you.

As you patiently wait to feel the energy waves, you might evaluate the sensation on a moment-to-moment basis. Do the energy waves seem constant? Do the waves vary from instant to instant? Is the wind steady; or does it gust periodically, bringing new opportunities to you?

Moreover, do you hear music or divine sounds, as your focused consciousness tunes into the cosmic consciousness inside you and all around you? Is there energy in nature that you did not previously recognize or acknowledge?

EXERCISE: *"Tree Energy Exchange"*

NEEDED:
1. Loose-fitting clothing, ideally with your shoes removed.
2. Outdoor setting.
3. A tree that you can approach.

DIRECTIONS:

Would you like to experience an energy exchange with a tree? Anyone can do that. Simply put yourself in the right state of mind with an open, sharing attitude and then approach the tree reverently.

Ask the tree if you can share your energy with it in love. You can do this verbally or in silent thoughts. While trees don't have verbal communication with us, they can speak to us silently. Listen for a response. Trees are always open to giving, if our hearts are pure and open.

Wrap your arms around the tree and place the palms of both hands squarely on the base of the tree. Project healing energy to the tree is whatever colors of light energy feel appropriate to you. Trees love green, of course, but will gratefully accept all positive healing energy that you send—even white light or a kaleidoscope of colored light.

When you are finished projecting healing energy to the tree, remain in place. Thank the tree. Now wait for the tree's response again. Most likely, you will receive a warm, tingling sensation from the tree. This is the powerful, healing energy of the tree directed now at you.

Typically, you will receive words of advice or comments from the tree, as well. Trees speak softly in profound, simply truths. They can tell you something about nature or the natural landscape that they oversee. Trees are very wise and very giving guardians of the earth. They process light energy as naturally as we breathe. Thank the tree again.

EXERCISE: *"Petting a Dog or Cat"*

NEEDED:
1. Loose-fitting clothing, ideally with shoes removed.
2. A dog or cat that is comfortable in your presence.

3. A mat or pad for the pet to recline upon during the session.
4. A quiet, isolated room is best.

DIRECTIONS:

Begin by comforting the pet and assuring it that you care for it and will do it no harm. Use a soothing, soft voice.

Then enter a state of heightened consciousness while sitting or squatting quietly next to the pet. Tune out external and internal distractions and reach that quiet, still spot deep inside you. This is where spirit resides in harmony with your energy body.

Move very slowly and deliberately toward the pet, assuring it of your gentleness and friendliness. Begin to pet the animal softly and lovingly with your right hand.

Consciously project energy through your outstretched hand. You will know that you are successful in projecting energy through your hand when you feel a warmth or tingling sensation in this hand. Send whatever energy seems appropriate.

If you establish telepathic communication with the pet, perhaps it will tell you what sort of energy it needs or what area needs rejuvenation. The anatomy of a dog or cat is similar to that of people. Their chakra system is nearly identical to ours, too. Just send the energy that you sense will most help the pet. If you receive no telepathic instructions from the pet and cannot determine its specific needs, simply send white light, soothing blue light, or even a kaleidoscope of colored light energy. The animal will gratefully receive and process all of the energy that you give it.

Remember that dogs, cats, and horses communicate telepathically in symbols, not words. They will send you images to convey their thoughts or feelings. Be receptive to this possibility in your heightened state of consciousness. You should have greater receptivity in this heightened state.

Thank the animal and wait with both of your hands resting gently upon the animal's back or wherever seems most comfortable for both of you.

Most likely, the animal will begin to send healing energy to you in return. This will last for as long as the animal decides, so wait patiently and respectfully to accept everything the animal wants to give you. Then thank the animal again.

EXERCISE—*"Personal Preparation"*

NEEDED:
1. Loose fitting clothes, shoes removed
2. Straight-back chair.
3. Quiet, isolated room is best.

DIRECTIONS:
Sit erect in the chair with your feet firmly planted on the group. Clear your mind of all internal and external distractions and consciously begin to put your physical body to rest, beginning with toes and working your way to the top of your head. Find that quiet still point deep within you—a place of tranquility and inner focus. Cease all internal dialogue and thought. Still your lower, analytical mind.

Soon you will begin to see a clear, blank slate in your mind's eye. Do not analyze it, but simple focus upon it. As your analytical mind or brain becomes numb and immobile, your higher consciousness becomes activated. This is your higher mind and the seat of heightened awareness. You will begin to sense this heightened awareness, as your higher consciousness races a mile a minute and you feel more totally awake and alive than you have felt before.

Begin to rub the palms of your hands together softly and slowly, conscious of the energy that extends from your hands. Focus on projecting your energy through your hands with conscious intent.

Now slowly separate your hands a few inches, so that the palms are facing each other but not touching. Sense the energy that passes between your two hands. Feel a tingling sensation or warmth. Pull the hands farther apart to feel the energy connection at a distance. Then bring the hands closer together. Become sensitized to the reality of energy in your body and your ability to project this energy in a way that can be felt.

EXERCISE—*"Preparing a Healing Subject"*

NEEDED:
1. Loose-fitting clothes, shoes removed.
2. Two straight-back chairs.
3. A patient intake form of sheet of paper with pen or pencil for writing.
4. A quiet, isolated room is ideal.

DIRECTIONS:

Begin by asking your healing subject to answer intake questions on a prepared form or else respond to your verbal questions on a blank piece of paper. Questions should include name, age, health concerns, health history, medication, noted symptoms, and family health history that might be pertinent. Ask what seems to be the problem, what parts of the body seem to be ailing, and whether personal energy seems low in any area of the body. If you do not have a prepared intake form with such questions, then perhaps you could simply interview your healing subject and record response yourself on a blank sheet of paper. A clip board would prove helpful, since you can sit in chairs and chat comfortable without going to a table for a writing surface.

Then direct your healing subject to sit erect in the chair, facing you in your chair with feet firmly anchored on the ground. Guide your subject into a state of heightened consciousness, as outlined above. Tell your friend to tune out all internal and external distractions and cease all thought. Now is the time to clear the mind and find a quiet, still point deep inside. Direct your subject to visualize a clean, blank slate in the mind's eye, without analyzing it. Have your subject consciously put the body to sleep, beginning with the toes and working all the way up to the head. Allow time for your healing subject to reach a personal state of heightened consciousness.

Now follow the same directions yourself, entering a personal state of heightened consciousness, as you face your healing subject in your own chair.

You are now ready to begin reading your healing subject's energy field as a prelude to chakra healing.

EXERCISE—"Reading the Aura"

NEEDED:
1. Loose-fitting clothes, with shoes removed.
2. Two straight-back chairs.
3. A quiet, isolated room is ideal.
4. Preparation, as described in the above exercises.

DIRECTIONS:

Face your healing subject and begin to scan the area just beyond the head and shoulders by shifting your eyes a little to the left. Do not stare directly at any area, but allow your eyes to become a little out of focus. It is important that you do not analyze or think about what see in depth, but simply take it all in. You are not seeing with your eyes directly, but simply using your physical eyes as a guide. In truth, you are divining or scrying. You are seeing in part with your mind's eye.

At first you may see white clusters of light that hang over the head and shoulders of your healing subject. Get a feel for the shape and contour of this energy field. Notice where it is located.

Now shift your eyes even a little more out of focus and begin to take the energy inside your mind's eye for a more critical examination. Do not think about the energy. Avoid thought or words inside your head. Simply focus on the energy inside your mind's eye and begin to sense the color values of the energy field.

Slowly the energy field will begin to assume color values inside your mind's eye. You might note a little patch of yellow colored light here and a little patch of green colored light there, for example. Do not look for anything specifically. Just allow the light to identify itself inside your mind's eye. You are seeing internally.

Once you have established some sense of color values to the energy field of the healing subject in front of you, return your gaze more directly to the subject. Begin to establish the extent of each color's pattern and area within the whole energy field. For example, where does the yellow light begin and end? What typical chakra colors are absent from the visible aura?

After you have scanned the aura thoroughly, then refer to your patient intake notes to determine what chakras seem to be stressed or challenged. Does the aura indicate a sufficient energy buildup of the chakra light energy colors most needed for healing? Does the aura indicate healing underway? What color of healing energy light is most needed to stimulate the challenged chakras and supplement their self-rejuvenation within your healing subject?

EXERCISE—*"Body Scan"*

NEEDED:
1. Loose-fitting clothes, with shoes removed.
2. Two straight-back chairs.
3. A quiet, isolated room is ideal.
4. Preparation in the above manner, including aura reading.

DIRECTIONS:

After reading the aura of your healing subject, you can get out of your chair and slowly walk to the back of your seated friend. Do not speak, unless necessary. It might be possible to explain briefly that you will do a simple energy scan now and assure your friend that it will not involve any touching or prove bothersome in any way.

Standing behind your friend, bring your hands together within about six inches, as though clutching an invisible ball near the top of the sphere. Consciously focus your intent on the energy to your hands to project energy. .Do not proceed until you sense the energy buildup in your hands. If you have trouble feeling any such energy buildup, then slowly rub your hands together and measure the energy ball that you have created by parting your hands six inches apart again. You might need to concentrate on centering yourself and focusing your intent to project the energy in a way that you can measure in such an energy ball.

Once you sense that you are projecting energy from your hands, withdraw the energy and refocus your intent on receiving energy signals in your hands. The first step of projecting energy from your hands helps you to sensitize your hands to energy. Now you will focus on scanning your healing subject to receive energy impulse from the subject's body.

Begin with your cupped hands on either side of your friend's head. Focus your attention on receiving energy impulses, as you scan for anomalies in the energy field. You will sense these anomalies in your hands and deep inside you as hot spots, cold spots, tingling feelings, or perhaps hollow feelings. Pause in place to determine whether you receive any such signals as indications of energy anomalies. Slowly work you way down the head, shoulders, arms, torso, and legs of your healing subject, pausing every few inches to determine whether you sense any anomalies in your cupped hands. Always face the palms of your hands to the subject's body.

Once you have finished your energy body scan from the back side, scan the front of your friend's body in the same manner.

If your efforts produced no indications of anomalies, then you might want to repeat the process from the back and front again.

Once you have completed your scan, sit down quietly in the chair and meditate on your findings. What chakras seemed to have energy anomalies? What colored light energy is associated with the chakra or chakras that seemed to be challenged? Does this fit or supplement the information you received in your aura reading?

Do you have a clear idea now what color or colors of light energy your friend requires for self-rejuvenation, based on troubled spots detected in your body scan and colors represented in the aura?

EXERCISE—"With a Second Healer"

NEEDED:
1. Loose-fitting clothing, with shoes removed.
2. 3 straight-back chairs.
3. An experienced assistant to work with you and your healing subject.
4. Preparation of all three participants to enter state of heightened awareness.

DIRECTIONS:
After you have read the aura of your healing subject, have your assistant also read the subject's aura. You should both remain in chairs, facing the healing subject and proceeding with as little discussion or movement as possible. Ideally, you would discuss your plans ahead of time. After you have both read the subject's aura with regard to health concerns, compare your impressions with your assistant. (Of course, this requires an assistant who is capable of aura reading.)

You might also have your assistant scan the healing subject's body with hands just off the surface of the body to determine possible anomalies in the energy flow. In this case, you will both need to rise from your chair and stand beside the healing subject. Do this one at a time, however, with one healer remaining in the chair. Move slowly and quietly. Once you have both scanned the back and front of the subject's body thoroughly, you can compare your impressions of the energy scans to determine which chakras are most challenged. When you have made this determination, you can project light energy to the subject in the color that is most associated with the stressed chakra to stimulate self-regeneration.

EXERCISE—"Projecting Light Energy"

NEEDED:
1. Loose-fitting clothing, with shoes removed.
2. Two straight-back chairs.
3. A quiet, isolated room is ideal.
4. Preparation by entering heightened awareness and energy scan to determine needs.

DIRECTIONS:

Once you have scanned your healing subject's energy field to determine which chakra needs support, simply determine which color of light energy is most associated with that challenged chakra. Remember, root chakra is red. Sacral chakra is orange. The solar plexus chakra is yellow. The heart chakra is green. The throat chakra is blue. The brow chakra is indigo. The crown chakra is violet.

Project the specific color of light that will stimulate and supplement the challenged chakra. Picture this color of light in your mind's eye and focus your intent with the full power of your will to project this color to the ailing chakra. In a real sense, you are manifesting color and sending it in a thought form. Your thought form is energy, encapsulated in this case with the color of light most required for self-rejuvenation by the stressed chakra. Creatively visualize the color and then visualize the color being absorbed by your ailing friend in the transfer process.

You must be in a meditative state of heightened consciousness to manifest and project energy in a thought form. If you sense that this is not working, then you should make another effort to center yourself and enter a proper state of heightened awareness.

EXERCISE—*"Projecting Sound Energy"*

NEEDED:
1. Loose-fitting clothes, with shoes removed.
2. Two straight-back chairs.
3. A quiet, isolated room is ideal.
4. Preparation to include energy scan.
5. A pitch pipe, flute, or other instrument might prove helpful.

DIRECTIONS:

You can also stimulate and supplement a challenged chakra by projecting the musical note that is most associated with the chakra in question. There are various approaches to this technique. You could use a pitch pipe, a flute, or another musical instrument to project the precise note that resonates harmonically with the chakra in need.

Energy is carried in sound waves just as effectively as it is carried in light waves. The frequency of the waves determines the pitch of a sound wave or the color of a light vibration. Consequently, the note middle C corresponds to red colored light. Either will stimulate and supplement the energy most associated with the root chakra. Similarly, the note D will stimulate the sacral chakra. The note E will stimulate the solar plexus chakra. The note F will stimulate the heart chakra. The G note will stimulate the throat chakra. The brow chakra can be stimulated by the A note. And the note B will stimulate the crown chakra.

These notes harmonically resonate with the natural energy of specific chakras in this fashion. In harmonically resonating with the energy of these corresponding chakras, they strengthen the structural integrity of the chakra as a swirling vortex of psychic energy.

Instead of a pitch pipe or other instrument to strike the proper note to stimulate a specific chakras, you might vocally sing the note. Of course, you would need to have a good sense of pitch to do this vocally. If you are unsure of your sense of pitch, use a musical instrument. And if you cannot pick out these seven notes on an instrument, use a pitch pipe. Remember to hold the note as long as possible and then repeat the note over and over.

Another approach would be to manifest the note inside you and transfer this sound in a thought form. This technique can be used in distant healing to send healing sound energy anywhere to anyone in need. Even if you are chanting the note aloud, you should employ thought power to creatively visualize the energy reaching the ailing chakra and being effectively absorbed and processed by the chakra.

EXERCISE—*"Distant Healing"*

NEEDED:
1. Loose-fitting clothes, with shoes removed
2. A quiet, isolated room is ideal.
3. Preparation to put yourself in a state of heightened awareness.

DIRECTIONS:
Visualize an ailing friend or loved one who needs your help. It is best to discuss your attempt to send healing energy with your friend in advance, so that you receive permission to do so. On the other hand, perhaps you already know that your help would be appreciated. Picture this friend in your mind's eye and meditate on contacting this friend. Make a conscious intent with the full power of your will to send healing energy to this friend, as soon as you reach a state of heightened awareness.

Now center yourself and put yourself into a state of higher consciousness. You can do this standing up or in a chair. The important thing is that you consciously put your body to sleep, while staying keenly alert. It might prove easier at first to do this exercise in a chair or even reclining on your bed.

Once you feel numb all over, your higher consciousness should activate. You will feel extremely alert and awake, despite the physical numbness of your physical body. When you reach this state, all thoughts and distractions should leave you. You will reach a still point deep within you.

Now picture a blank slate in your mind's eye. Slowly allow the image of your friend to fill this blank slate, so your entire focus is solely on this friend. You have carried with you the conscious intent to send healing energy to this friend. If you know the chakra area of your friend that needs an energy boost, send that color of light energy to your friend to assist in healing. Or perhaps you can send the musical note that resonates with the chakra in question. Simply focus on the image of your friend and project this healing note. Your energized thought form will reach your friend to assist in healing wherever your friend may be. You can encapsulate your thought form with light energy or sound energy that you manifest and project with your thought form. Your healing thought form will reach your friend anywhere like a magnet, because you have a bond through karmic attraction. This involves electromagnetism, the essence of our being and all life that is known to us.

Finally, picture your friend actually receiving your healing thought forms and absorbing the energy that you have sent. Visualize your friend processing this healing energy and beginning to rejuvenate naturally.

EXERCISE: "Healing a Pet"

As we have seen, there is a natural energy bond between people and their pets. We can exchange energy with our pets in much the same way that we can share energy with people to assist in natural rejuvenation. Minor differences involve how we treat pets during chakra healing sessions. There will be no interview or intake session, unless you can fill in the blanks yourself or talk to somebody who knows something about the pet's health condition. Also, you can't follow usual procedure in directing a pet to center itself and enter a state of heightened awareness, while seated in a chair. On the other hand, you can speak softly and lovingly to the pet to assure it that you are going to help it feel better. You can ask it to relax. Fortunately, most animals find it easier to enter a state of heightened awareness than most people, so you won't need to concern yourself about centering the pet prior to your session. Animals, such as our dogs and cats, walk closely with nature and live in the moment.

NEEDED:
1. Loose-fitting clothing, ideally with shoes removed.
2. A dog or cat that is comfortable in your presence.
3. A mat or blanket for the pet to recline on the floor.
4. A quiet, isolated room is ideal.

DIRECTIONS:

Once you have assured the animal verbally and pet it to show that you are friendly, put yourself into a heightened state of consciousness by centering yourself and tuning out all distraction. Focus on your conscious intent to heal this animal by determining its needs and sharing your energy to help it regenerate.

Allow the pet to recline on the mat or wherever it seems most comfortable in the room. You might need to move around to accommodate the pet in whatever position it seems most comfortable.

Read the pet's aura to determine what colors of light energy are most present in its aura and which are absent. Then scan the pet slowly and gently with your hands near its body to sense any energy anomalies that might be present in the chakra system of the pet.

Once you determine what color of light energy would be most helpful to the pet, based on energy shortages in the chakra system, focus your thought form to project this color of light energy to the pet. Aim it directly at the chakra that is most in need, the chakra that is primarily associated with that particular color of light energy.

Visualize the light energy being absorbed and processed effectively by the pet's chakra. Visualize the natural rejuvenation process beginning to work within the pet.

Pet the animal gently on the head, ears, behind the shoulders, or whatever spot seems most comfortable for both of you.

In a soft and gentle voice thank the pet and wish it well.

EXERCISE: *"Healing a Plant"*

NEEDED:
1. Loose-fitting clothes, ideally with shoes removed.
2. A nearby plant that has a special connection to you.
3. A quiet atmosphere.

DIRECTIONS:
Approach the plant slowly and lovingly. Look at the plant and tell it that you will not harm it, but only want it to be healthy and thrive. You can say this in a thought form or say it aloud.

Prepare yourself by centering and entering a state of heightened consciousness, with the focused intent to project healing energy to the plant. Clear your mind, so that all you see is a blank slate in your mind's eye. Now let the image of the plant fill that slate. Visualize the plant in your mind's eye. Picture it getting healthier.

Gaze at the plant and scan the energy field that surrounds it as an aura. Do you sense anything odd about the aura, such as a brown cloud, black cloud, or ragged energy field?

Now slowly walk to the plant and begin to scan the plants body with the palms of your hands just inches from the body of the plant. Scan the energy field of the entire plant, including all leaves and stems. Do you notice any anomalies?

Face the plant again and begin sending healing energy in whatever color of light seems appropriate to you. Green is a good healing color for a plant. So is white. Or you might do even better by sending a whole kaleidoscope of colored light in succession. The plant will take what it needs and process it for rejuvenation.

Lastly, you can approach the plant again and send energy from the palms of your hands in body energy work. Do not actually touch the leaves and stems of the plant, but maintain a distance of a couple of inches. Focus your intent on projecting healing energy in whatever color of light seems most appropriate. If your hands do not tingle or feel warm during this healing session, then take a moment to center yourself again and rub your hands together until you feel an energy buildup in your hands. This is usually experienced as warmth or pulsing feeling in the hands, as they are ready to project healing energy.

It is helpful during body healing work with your hands to visualize the color of light energy that you want to project and then manifest that color of light in your mind's eye. Visualize the colored light leaving you and entering the plant. You are manifesting energy inside you and transferring it to the plant. To complete the creative visualization, picture the plant absorbing and processing the light energy that you send to it. Visualize it beginning to rejuvenate.

Bibliography

Abendroth, Jack H. *The Book of Light*. Philadelphia, PA: Xlibris Corporation, 2000.

Andrews, Ted. *How to See and Read the Aura*. St. Paul, Minn.: Llewellyn Publications, 1991.

Bailey, Alice. *The Light of the Soul*. New York: Lucis Publishing Company. 1955.

Besant, Annie. *Thought Power*. Wheaton, Ill.: Theosophical Publishing House, 1998.

Braschler, Von. *Conversations with the Dream Mentor*. St. Paul, Minn.: Llewellyn Publications, 2003.

——— *Natural Pet Healing*. Lakeville, Minn.: Galde Press, 2003.

Brennan, Barbara Ann. *Hands of Light: A Guide to Healing through the Human Energy Field*. New York: Bantam Doubleday Dell, 1988.

Campbell, Don. *The Roar of Silence: Healing Powers of Breath, Tone & Chant*. Wheaton, Ill.: Theosophical Publishing House, 1989.

Carter, Mildred, and Tammy Weber. *Body Reflexology: Healing at your Fingertips*. West Nyack, NY: Parker Publishing Company, 1994.

Choa Kok Sui. *The Ancient Science & Art of Pranic Healing.* Quezon City, Metro City, Philippines: Institute for Inner Studies, 1987.

——, *Pranic Psychotherapy.* York Beach, Maine: Samuel Weiser, Inc., 1993.

Dale, Cyndi. *New Chakra Healing.* St. Paul, Minn.: Llewellyn Publishing, 1996.

Godwin, Joscelyn. *Harmonies of Heaven and Earth: The Spiritual Dimensions of Music.* Rochester, Vermont: Inner Traditions International, Ltd., 1987.

Hay, Louise. *Heal Your Body.* Carlesbad, Calif.: Hay House, 1988.

Kreiger, Dolores. *Living the Therapeutic Touch: Healing as a Lifestyle.* New York: Dodd, Mead & Company, 1987.

——, *The Therapeutic Touch: How to Use your Hands to Help or to Heal.* New York: Prentice Hall Press, 1979.

——, Erik Peper, and Sonia Ancoli. "Therapeutic Touch: Searching for Evidence of Physiological Change," *The Theosophical Research Journal,* December, 1986.

Karagulla, Shafica, and Dora Van Gelder Kunz. *The Chakras & the Human Energy Fields.* Wheaton, Ill.: Theosophical Publishing House, 1998.

Kawalski, Gary. *The Souls of Animals.* Walpole, NH: Stillpoint Publishing, 1991.

Kunz, Dora. *Spiritual Aspects of the Healing Arts.* Wheaton, Ill.: Theosophical Publishing House, 1985.

———, and Erik Peper. "Fields and their Clinical Implications," *American Theosophist*, Nov. 1982, Jan. 1983, June 1983, Aug. 1984, Sept. 1984, and Nov. 1985 (six parts)

Lansdown, Zachary F. *Ray Methods of Healing.* York Beach, Maine: Samuel Weiser, Inc. 1993.

Leadbeater, Charles W. *The Chakras.* Wheaton, Ill.: Theosophical Publishing House, 1997.

Lingerman, Hal. *The Healing Energies of Music.* Wheaton, Ill.: Theosophical Publishing House, 1995.

Mathews, John. *Healing the Wounded King: Soul Work and the Quest for the Grail.* Rockport, MA: Element Books, 1997.

Newton, Michael. *Journey of Souls.* St. Paul, Minn.: Llewellyn Publications, 1999.

Puharich, Andrija. *Uri: The Original and Authorized Biography of Uri Geller—The Man who Baffled Scientists.* London: W. H. Allen, 1974.

Ray, Barbara. *The Reiki Factor.* St. Petersburg, Florida: Radiance Associates, 1986.

Rifkin, Jeremy. *Entropy: Into the Greenhouse World*. New York: Bantam Books, 1989.

Satchadananda, Sri S. *The Yoga Sutras of Patanjali*. Buckingham, Virginia: Integral Yoga Distribution, 1990.

Smith, Penelope. *Animal Talk: Interspecies Telepathic Communication*. Point Reyes Station, CA: Pegasus Publications, 1996.

———, *Animals...Our Return to Wholeness*. Point Reyes Station, CA: Pegasus Publications, 1993.

Steiner, Lee R. *Psychic Self-Healing for Psychological Problems*. Englewood Cliff, NJ: Prentice-Hall, Inc., 1977.

Stone, Robert B. *The Secret Life of Your Cells*. Atglen, PA: Whitford Press, 1989.

Tellington-Jones, Linda, and Sybil Taylor. *The Tellington Touch: A Revolutionary Natural Method to Train and Care for your Favorite Animal*. New York: Penguin Putnam, 1995.

Tessman, Diane. *Seven Rays of the Healing Millennium*. New Brunswick, NJ: Inner Light Publications, 1998.

Tompkins, Peter, and Christopher Bird. *The Secret Life of Plants*. New York: Harper & Row, Publishers, Inc., 1989.

———, *Secrets of the Soil*. Anchorage, Alaska: Earthpulse Press Incorporated, 1998.

Tyson, Donald. *Scrying for Beginners: Tapping into the Supersensory Powers of your Subconscious.* St. Paul, Minn.: Llewellyn Publications, 1997.

Webster, Richard. *Aura Reading for Beginners.* St. Paul, Minn.: Llewellyn Publications, 1998.

Wood, Ernest. *The Seven Rays.* Wheaton, Ill.: Theosophical Publishing House, 1972.

Index

Abendroth, Jack 218
Active concerns 26
Additional treatment 187
Adrenal gland 27, 172
Adventure 34, 159
Allopathic medicine 42, 55
Altered chakras 186
Amethyst 103
Anemia 27
Anger 31, 41, 172
Apollo 150, 154
Aquarius 36
Aries 29
Arms 32, 53, 60, 71, 74, 172, 196, 199, 201, 208
Arthurian legend 154
Artists 34
Assessing 57, 61, 74, 145
Assistant 177, 209
Asthma 30
Astringent 33
Attraction 30, 90-92, 115, 213
Auras . . 10, 14-17, 19-22, 26, 27, 40, 47, 62, 83, 94, 107, 112, 121,
137, 177, 178, 190
Auric field 39, 40
B note 95, 97

Background tools 71
Badly injured 187
Bailey, Alice 218
Balance 13, 28, 30, 32, 150, 172, 188
Battery 21, 22, 91, 117-119, 144, 153
Birth signs 29
Black cloud 22, 23, 137, 189, 216
Bliss 35, 172
Blockages of energy 57
Blood diseases 27
Bloodstone 103
Blue . . . 15, 18, 19, 21, 32-34, 40, 41, 47, 71, 72, 77-79, 83, 87, 95,
133, 169, 171, 186, 189, 190, 195, 202, 210
Body language 62, 166, 197
Book of Light 195, 218
Bronchial 33, 172
Bronchitis 30
Brow 34, 40, 79, 97, 109, 171, 172, 210, 211
Brown cloud 21, 216
Burns 33
Calming 33, 87, 126, 166, 189
Camera 12, 18, 54, 120, 123, 145
Cancer 36, 162, 178
Candles 29-32, 35, 71, 95
Capricorn 32, 33
Case file 68, 140, 145
Cathars 195
Cats 11, 29, 61, 112, 166, 168-172, 202, 214
Causal body 40, 44, 45, 47
Centaur 154, 156

Centaurus 155
Chakra chart 83, 84
Chakras . 9, 10, 12, 13, 18, 19, 23, 28, 36, 38, 41, 48, 50, 63, 64, 71,
    76-81, 83, 91, 94, 95, 106, 107, 111, 112, 114, 118-123, 128-
        139, 143, 147, 148, 165, 168, 169, 171, 174, 177-179, 183,
            186, 187, 190, 194, 206-209, 211, 212, 219, 220
Changeable 32
Charging 102, 136
Charming 34
Charting progress 6, 140
Chest 32, 71, 74, 92, 171, 172
Chiron 154-156, 158, 161
Christians 161, 195
Church 14, 15, 195
Circular energy 34
Circulation problems 27
Circulatory system 32, 172
Citrine 103
Clairaudients 36
Closed systems 197, 198
Colic 33
Color therapy 28, 29, 32, 33, 94, 95
Color values 206
Communication 33, 125, 167, 172, 201, 202, 221
Compassion 34, 169, 172
Confidence 31, 70, 177, 178
Congestion 59
Consecrating 102
Constipation 27, 31
Cool vibration 33

Corona discharge 56
Creative visualization 22, 83, 87, 91, 92, 98, 99, 104, 107, 109,
110, 126, 136, 144, 177, 182, 183, 185, 217
Creativity 31
Crown chakra . . . 35, 40, 42, 58, 71, 79, 95, 97, 103, 169, 171, 172, 210, 211
Cuts 33
D note 97
Death 19, 22, 23, 63, 64, 137, 155, 161, 188, 189
Developmental disorders 34
Devotion 33
Diabetes 31
Diatonic music scale 28, 31, 192
Difficult cases 178
Digestive system 31, 103
Distant healing 91, 92, 212
Distractions . . 53, 70, 72, 82, 85, 103, 108, 149, 177, 199, 200, 202, 203, 205, 213
Divination 48-50, 57, 107, 108, 146
Divine essence 39, 40, 45, 46, 111, 112, 129, 139, 195
Divine Spark 25, 112, 189, 193
Dogs 11, 29, 61, 108, 112, 166, 168-172, 174, 202, 214
Dream work 35
Dream world 157
Dreaming 34, 172
Dynamos 24, 28, 44, 56, 76, 115, 118, 131, 183
Dyspepsia 31
E note 97
Ears 33, 149, 171, 172, 215
Eckenkar 195

Ego ... 148
Electromagnetic field ... 119
Emotional body ... 39, 40, 43-45, 58, 111, 125
Ending the session ... 74
Energy .. 5, 6, 9-16, 18-44, 46-50, 53-74, 76-139, 141-154, 160, 162, 163, 165, 167-219
Energy wave ... 26
Epilepsy ... 30
Etheric layer ... 43
Ethics ... 115
Europe ... 195
Excessive energy ... 135, 180
Exercises ... 6, 199, 205
Exhausting ... 67
Expressiveness ... 33, 172
Eye problems ... 34
Eyes ... 11, 17, 18, 20, 22, 34, 45, 48, 49, 54, 55, 60, 62, 82, 85, 93, 94, 107-109, 139, 144, 168, 171, 172, 190, 206
F note ... 96, 97
Feedback response ... 101
Feet .. 27, 38, 46, 52-54, 57, 59, 61, 70, 71, 125, 172, 176, 188, 203, 205
Fertility ... 32, 33
Fevers ... 33, 103
Finance ... 32
Flexible ... 32
Forehead ... 17, 34, 35, 92, 95, 171
Fortune ... 30
France ... 195

Frequency .. 26, 28, 30-33, 35, 65, 72, 84, 86, 94-96, 109, 113, 119, 183, 195, 211
G note 97, 211
Gall bladder 31, 172
Garden flowers 193
Gaze 17, 62, 63, 206, 216
Gemini 31
Giving 19, 32, 66, 71, 123, 198, 201
Godwin, Joscelyn 219
Goiter 33
Grail quest 159
Grave illness 63
Gray 63, 188, 190, 191
Greek mythology 154
Green 15, 18-21, 32, 33, 41, 63, 71, 72, 78, 79, 82, 87, 95, 133, 171, 189, 201, 206, 210, 216
Grieving 33, 172
Growth 32, 33, 47, 66, 96
Hands ... 11, 16, 22, 32, 36, 43, 53, 57-60, 66, 71, 76, 92, 100-102, 104, 109, 119-121, 123-125, 132, 134, 136, 138, 139, 146, 168-170, 172-174, 177, 178, 184, 186, 189, 190, 196, 197, 201, 203, 204, 207-209, 215, 216, 218, 219
Happiness 30
Harm 56, 87, 151, 202, 215
Harmonies of Heaven and Earth 219
Harmony 9, 11, 30, 32, 34, 96, 158, 202
Hay, Louise 219
Headaches 32, 34, 153
Healing with hands 100, 123
Health aura 63, 64, 101, 125, 130

Hearing problems	34
Heart	11, 32, 33, 41, 63, 79, 82, 87, 95-97, 103, 133, 169, 171, 172, 178, 181, 183, 199, 210, 211
Heart problems	32
Heightened consciousness	10-12, 17, 27, 37, 46, 53, 55, 59, 60, 71, 72, 74, 82, 83, 85, 90, 99, 106, 108, 109, 124, 125, 138, 142, 144, 147, 149, 166, 190, 199, 200, 202, 205, 210, 216
Herakles (Hercules)	155
Hero's journey	161
Higher awareness	17
Higher emotions	33, 172
Higher knowledge	35, 172
Higher mind	11, 17, 35, 45, 108, 177, 203
Higher self	45, 108, 129
Hippocratic Oath	150
Hoarseness	33
Holism	35, 172
Horses	29, 61, 112, 166, 168-172, 202
Houseplants	11, 78, 193
HU	195
Hurt	83, 151
Hydra	155
Imagination	34, 46, 172
Imbalance	13, 34, 134, 180, 185
Impossible	6, 62, 64, 182, 184, 186
Indigo	18, 34, 35, 40, 71, 72, 78, 79, 95, 133, 134, 171, 210
Individualized consciousness	39, 40, 45, 46
Intellectual	36

Intent 10, 21, 24, 29, 36, 44, 45, 70, 73, 82, 85, 90, 92, 98-102, 104, 107, 110, 114, 115, 149, 152, 173, 177, 181, 184, 204, 207, 208, 210, 212-214, 216
Internalize 190
Intonation 98-100
Intuitive ability 37
Jaundice 33
Jaw 33
Jesus 161
Journey of Souls 196, 220
Jump-start 22, 81, 117-119, 144, 153
Karen 16, 19, 20, 22
Kidneys 27, 29, 72, 172
Kindness 30
Kirlian photography 56, 102, 119-121, 173
Kronos 154
Laryngitis 33
Larynx 33
Laughter 31, 172
Legs 27, 61, 71, 74, 169, 172, 192, 208
Leo 30
Light . 11, 12, 14-19, 21, 23, 24, 26-36, 38, 39, 41, 47-49, 52, 54-56, 62, 63, 65, 71, 72, 76-83, 85-87, 89-91, 93-96, 98, 102, 104, 108, 109, 111-113, 115, 119, 122, 123, 126, 130, 131, 133-136, 139, 143-146, 149-151, 165, 169, 171, 172, 174, 177, 179, 183, 185, 186, 189, 190, 192-196, 201, 202, 206-211, 213, 215-218, 221
Light being 38, 65
Light energy ... 16, 18, 19, 28, 29, 31-36, 39, 47, 49, 54-56, 62, 63, 65, 72, 76-80, 83, 87, 89, 93-95, 98, 109, 111, 122, 123, 130,

> 131, 133-136, 139, 143, 145, 149-151, 165, 171, 172, 174, 177, 179, 183, 185, 190, 192, 201, 202, 207-210, 213, 215-217

Light of the soul 195, 218
Liver 31
Love feelings 41, 63
Loving 16, 32, 99, 170-172, 181, 183, 193, 196
Low energy 183
Lower mind 34, 44, 45, 108, 172
Luminous body 38
Luminous egg shell 47
Lungs 32, 33, 87, 133, 172
Lymph system 31
Magic 5, 9, 10, 19, 27, 30, 34, 35, 85, 107, 108, 113, 115
Magnets 101, 127, 179
Magus 182
Manifest . . . 16, 18, 36, 73, 86, 94, 98, 126, 135, 136, 143, 149, 182, 190, 193, 195, 210, 212, 213, 216
Meditation 10, 27, 37, 54, 68, 82, 92, 143, 149, 185, 199
Melancholy 35
Mental body 40, 44, 45, 78
Mental disorders 30, 34, 35, 44
Mental will 31, 172
Mentally intense 32
Middle Ages 195
Middle C 28, 72, 95-97, 192, 211
Mission-driven 32
Mouth 33, 100
Musical notes 95, 99, 194
Musicians 28

Natural light 26, 78, 151, 174
Natural magic 9, 10, 108, 113
Nature   . . .   9, 11, 13, 37, 41, 43-45, 48, 65, 66, 68, 76, 78, 113, 122, 123, 126, 156-158, 161, 162, 170, 172, 192, 200, 201, 214
Nerves 31, 133, 134
Nervous conditions 30, 35
Nervous system 34, 172
New Age 156
Newton, Michael 220
Non-physical seeing 62
Nurturers 36
Open systems 197, 198
Orange 18, 29, 30, 63, 71, 72, 78, 85, 95, 171, 210
Oregon 14, 15
Orientation 9, 10, 67, 70, 162, 166, 174
Outer shell 38, 39, 42
Overall good health 32
Overload 29, 57, 134, 135, 143, 180
Palpitation 33
Pancreas 31, 172
Paralysis 27
Paranjali 195
Parathyroid 33, 172
Patience 16, 92, 139, 148, 183, 186
Patient questionnaire 68
Perceval 159, 160, 162
Personality 34, 45, 172
Persuasion 31
Pets 6, 23, 61, 62, 76, 165-172, 174, 175, 180, 181, 187, 214
Philyra 154

Photography 12, 56, 77, 93, 102, 119-121, 173
Photosynthesis 78
Physical body . 10-12, 38-45, 47, 56, 58, 59, 62, 63, 78, 81, 93, 101,
    108, 109, 112, 120, 125, 129, 130, 139, 142, 163, 165, 169,
    174, 185, 189, 203, 213
Physical debility 27
Piety 35
Piezo-electric principle 193
Pineal gland 35, 172
Pink 15, 41
Pisces 31, 32
Pituitary gland 34, 109, 172
Plants . . . 6, 11, 76, 78, 120, 121, 137, 165, 172-175, 180, 181, 193,
    194, 216, 221
Pneumonia 34
Power . 22, 31, 35, 73, 77, 80, 86, 90, 91, 93, 98-102, 104, 107, 110,
    111, 113, 114, 117, 123, 131, 151, 172, 185, 192, 195, 210,
    212, 218
Power of will 73
Practical considerations 6, 176
Pranic healers 54
Preparation 31, 205, 207, 209-212
Protective 33, 170
Psychic . 11, 16, 17, 27, 30, 31, 33, 35, 37-39, 41, 43-45, 47, 49, 54,
    79, 80, 89, 96, 109, 118, 121, 194, 211, 221
Psychic power 35
Psychological states 120
Psychometry 57, 89, 109
Quartz crystal 103, 193
Radiate . . . 11, 12, 18, 19, 25, 26, 40, 46, 47, 55, 128, 190, 194, 195

Reading . 1, 5, 6, 9, 10, 16, 17, 19, 20, 22, 24-27, 37, 40, 47-49, 52-54, 56-58, 62, 67, 82, 83, 89, 93, 104, 108, 109, 128, 130, 131, 136, 140, 143, 153, 167, 177-179, 182, 189, 192, 197, 205, 207-209, 222

Red 18, 27-29, 32, 40, 41, 71, 72, 78, 81, 85, 95, 103, 133, 136, 171, 192, 210, 211

Red agate 103
Red blood cells 28
Reformers 36
Rejuvenation ... 6, 22, 56, 83, 87, 98, 100, 103, 105-108, 113, 114, 117, 118, 122, 146, 148, 151, 178, 183, 186, 187, 197, 202, 207, 208, 210, 214-216

Repeat treatments 146
Reproductive organs 28
Respiratory system 33, 172
Sagittarius 34
Saturn 155
Scanning 5, 16, 26, 53, 57-61, 67, 100, 101, 108, 136, 169, 178, 179, 208

Scorpio 29
Selecting colors 36
Self-discovery 153, 161
Self-healing 24, 53, 56, 105, 121, 143, 185, 221
Self-rejuvenation .. 6, 56, 83, 87, 98, 100, 105, 107, 113, 114, 117, 118, 122, 146, 151, 183, 186, 187, 207, 208, 210

Sense of smell 36
Serenity 33
Seven rays 18, 23, 24, 41, 55, 65, 78, 221, 222
Shamanic healers 157

Sharing 15, 66, 67, 114, 115, 126, 127, 153, 156, 175, 181, 187, 194, 197, 198, 201, 214
Shifted eyes 17, 62
Sincerity 33
Skin abrasion 33
Solar plexus 31, 40, 78, 82, 95, 97, 103, 171, 172, 210, 211
Soothing ... 32, 33, 61, 72, 87, 97, 99, 133, 150, 186, 189, 190, 202
Sore throat 33
Soul 35, 42, 46, 81, 111, 154, 157-162, 172, 194-196, 218, 220
Sound energy 72, 80, 89, 95-98, 111, 194, 212, 213
Speech problems 33
Spinal column 27, 172
Spine 27, 60, 81, 101, 166, 169, 171
Spirit body 38, 46, 58, 93, 103, 109, 189
Spirit to spirit 65, 114, 137
Spiritual bliss 35
Spirituality 35, 47
Squirming 168
Stimulating ... 6, 27, 30, 90, 105, 117-119, 122, 129, 186, 187, 194
Stomach 31, 100, 172
Stone, Robert 221
Stones 102, 103, 193
Stress responses 27, 172
Subtle bodies 5, 10-12, 19, 38-43, 45-47, 78, 81, 107, 111, 112, 120, 125, 129, 130, 142, 163, 165
Sunlight 17, 62, 78, 122, 123, 172, 175
Superman 182
Survival 27, 172
Swirling vortexes 79, 131
Symbiotic relationship 170

235

Symptoms . . 25, 42, 50, 51, 69, 70, 82, 128, 131, 140, 167, 176, 204
Techniques 5, 89, 99, 104
Third eye 17, 35, 50, 54, 62, 73, 79, 108, 109
Thought forms . . . 73, 90-95, 99, 109-111, 114, 125, 126, 144, 166, 167, 170, 171, 174, 177, 213
Thought power . . 73, 90, 91, 93, 102, 104, 107, 110, 111, 123, 212, 218
Three-ring binder 141
Thymus 32, 79, 82, 87, 172
Tingling . . . 57, 59, 71, 101, 102, 124, 125, 169, 173, 201, 202, 204, 208
Tonsils 33
Transformation . . 9, 19, 23, 32, 35, 55, 85, 107, 110-112, 135, 147, 172, 183
Trauma 50, 80, 81, 118, 131-133, 150, 152, 182, 185, 186
Travel 12, 31, 45, 46, 92, 93, 185
Truth 9, 11, 22, 23, 33, 45, 47, 112, 131, 196, 206
Understanding 33, 83, 122, 135, 162, 163, 172, 197
Upper abdomen 31, 172
Uranus 155
Urinary tract 28
Versatile 32
Vibrational energy 29
Vibrational quality 100
Violet 18, 27, 35, 36, 40, 71, 72, 78, 79, 95, 103, 171, 210
Virgo 31
Visionary thinking 34, 172
Vitalizing 27
Vocal 33, 167, 172
Water 11, 17, 65, 77, 102-104, 108, 154, 175

Wellness 32, 87
Wholeness 10, 38, 39, 156, 159, 160, 162, 163, 221
Will to live 27, 114, 115, 172
Wisdom 23, 34, 156, 160, 172, 195
Wonder Woman 182
Wounded healer 6, 153-158, 160-163
Yellow .. 12, 18, 21, 31, 32, 40, 71, 72, 78, 82, 85, 95, 171, 206, 210
Yoga Sutras 195, 221
Zeus 154, 155

Printed in the United States
38588LVS00005B/238-243